Coming Alive At 55

Let Me Show You How To Sleep Your Way To Great Health Now!!

Dr. M.D. Brown, 1st.

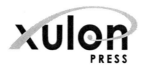

Copyright © 2008 by Dr. M.D. Brown, 1st.

Coming Alive at 55!!!
Let Me Show You How To
Sleep Your Way To Great Health Now!!
by Dr. M.D. Brown, 1st.

Printed in the United States of America

ISBN 978-1-60477-715-4

All rights reserved solely by the author. The author guarantees all contents are original and do not infringe upon the legal rights of any other person or work. No part of this book may be reproduced in any form without the permission of the author. The views expressed in this book are not necessarily those of the publisher.

Unless otherwise indicated, Bible quotations are taken from The King James Version, Copyright © 1909 by Oxford Press Inc., and the The New King James Version, Copyright © 1997 by Word Publishing, and The New American Standard Bible, Copyright © 1960 by Harvest House Publishers. Definitions were obtained from the Merriam-Webster's online dictionary and Bible. The word Vintaged from Julie Guardado. References to Elvis Presley are from the Elvis Presley website. Matt Wong's article was from ESPN.com. Kathleen Brown material is from her upcoming book to be named later.

www.xulonpress.com

It's Never Too Late To Start And It's Always Too Early To Quit!!

As a fine wine, you can get better with age!!
 Older things, if they are well preserved, tend to increase in Value!!! They Become Vintaged!
This book will show you in four easy steps:
How valuable you are and how to get this value out of you
How to run to your successes and not away from them.

Dr. M. D. Brown, *1st. Was told after he had been in a car wreck at the age of 51 that he would never run again!! He was also told that he would never jump or do any heavy lifting again!! Dr. M. D. Brown, 1st. was told he would need surgery to repair the herniated discs, and the synovial cyst on his spine!! He was told that there was no guarantee that this procedure would eliminate the pain in his back!!*

Through prayer, faith, determination, dedication and calling upon his over 40 years of physical fitness training, 24 years in the field of full potential development and 18 years in the Ministry; Dr. M. D. Brown, 1st. is running, jumping and lifting again!!! And the pain is gone!!!

Dr. M. D. Brown, 1st. Is the founder, President and Executive Director of M.D.B.1 ministries Inc., and a former Administrator. Dr. Brown has been helping individuals reach their full potential for 24 years. Dr. Brown holds B.A. degrees in theology, and biblical studies, an M.A. degree in biblical studies and a doctor of Ministry degree. Dr. Brown is also a certified marriage counselor & he is a former finance manager. He is a graduate of the Institute of Biblical Studies, recognized as a certified Sunday school developer and Christian leader by Moody Bible College. Dr. Brown is a former pastor. He is also the former host of the Midweek Message, and Sunday Mornings Study Christian radio programs.

Contents

Acknowledgments ix
Dedication xi
Preface xiii
Introduction xxi

Chapter   **Page**

1. The First Person of the Heavenly Trio: God the Father....25
2. The Second Person Of The Heavenly Trio:
     God The Son: 35
3. The Third Person Of the Heavenly Trio:
     God the Holy Spirit; 47
4. Holy Spirit Power 53
5. Spiritual Revelation for Deeper Understanding
     and Praise 57
6. Just Another Ordinary Day 65
7. Every Child Should Have Good Parents:
     Even Grown-Up Ones 71
8. Big Surprises Come in Small Packages 77
9. Hurry Up and Wait on God 85
10. Who are you going to straighten out? 93
11. Do You Really Want to Hear? Do You Really
      Want to See? 99
12. Too Mature to Be Fat! Too Vintaged To Look
      Like That! 109

13. Keep Your Eyes Open And Your Knees Bent! 117
14. A Little Bit Goes a Long Way 121
15. Everyone Catches & Goes Through Hell Sometimes! 131
16. You Can Fool Some People But You Can't Fool Mom! ... 141
17. What Did You Say Lord? Butts, Gut's And
    Gray Hairs? 151

Acknowledgments

To my mother Ella Brown, who has gone on to be with the Lord, and my father, Alonzo Brown. Your hard work and determination has always been the hallmark of our family's lives. I want to thank you for letting me know that no matter what, you must never give up and that you can achieve anything, if you work hard enough and have faith to achieve it.

To my dearly departed brother, Alonzo Brown Jr., thank you so very much for your talent, your sense of humor and your encouragement.

To my departed sister, Violet Brown, thank you for your wit, your comedy and your support. I miss you both so very much.

To my children, Camille, Mark 2nd. and Starla, may you continue to grow, develop and prosper into all that God wants you to become and may you be blessed beyond your wildest dreams.

To my grandchildren, Guy, Tyler, Adrian, Mark, Bennie & Tyrell, may you have uncommon wisdom and favor all your life.

To my brothers, James and Richard Brown, I want to thank you both for your intelligence, perseverance, dedication, laughter and loyalty. A baby brother could not ask for better examples then the two of you.

To my wife, Kathleen, my first lady and partner in this adventure we call life, thank you for bringing such great sunlight, rapture, courage, excitement and joy into my life. You were the missing piece of my perfect puzzle.

To my proof reading staff, Ethel Brown, Camille Brown & James A. Brown. Thank you for your dedicated service.

Dedication

To my grandmother and grandfather, Uzella and James Garrett, thank you for the soul food, and the spiritual food.

To my mother and father, Alonzo and Ella Brown, who taught me never to give up, never, never ever give up, thank you.

To my wife Kathleen, thank you for your understanding, patients, supports and encouragement during this exhilarating adventure.

To the "School Of Hard Knocks" and all of those bad circumstances and situations that are always prevalent in life. Thank you for the motivation, consistency and competition!!!

Preface

There are many things in life that are hard to live with. You may have a physical ailment, which you will have to live with for the rest of your life. To be faced with the fact that there is a loss in your family is an awful thing to live with. Someone in your family could have a disease, and they may be ill for the rest of their lives. Or a disease could take their life. Your children could be permanently impaired, and may need to have aid for as long as they may live.

You could experience great financial loss and lose everything that you have; you could lose your job, your business or your income and end up with nothing. Your husband or your wife could leave you and you could be thrown into a state of depression, despair and sorrow that you may think that you would never recover from. You could feel as if you could lose your mind!!

All of these issues are tremendous tragedies and there are many others that we can think of that have during the season that we were facing them seemed as if we would never recuperate from them. However, with the prayers, love, concern, understanding and the compassion of our loved ones, with faith determination, discipline, time and the grace of God. We are able to recover and continue on with our lives. It's wasn't easy but we made it.

We eventually do learn to live with that family loss, we learn to deal with the illness or the impairment. You overcome your financial loss, and you discover that there is more than one fish in the sea, and you do find another mate. Not to make light of these situations, but there is also another kind of tragedy that is also very difficult to live with.

That tragedy is living with unfulfilled expectations, undeveloped abilities or unused abilities. To have locked deep down inside of you something that you knew you could do but that you didn't do. To have something inside of you that you didn't get out of you.

To know you had these abilities and that had you developed them you could have really been something special. But for whatever reason, whether you were lazy lacked confidence lacked the knowledge or just didn't care or didn't realize the opportunity you were squandering, you never developed those abilities.

And this can happen to you no matter what your age or gender. That feeling of inadequacy of not being as good as you could be of not obtaining the level of power and skill that you know you should have.

To have locked inside of you a song, a song that you should have sang, but you didn't even go out for the choir. You knew you could sing and many people also told you that. With some training and hard work who knows how far you could have gone. Or a song that you should have written, but you didn't even put a pen or pencil to a piece of paper.

Or a play that you should have starred in, you seemed to be a natural born actress but you didn't even go out for the cast. Or that play that you could've written, but you didn't even attempt to write the first word.

Or, what about that job interview that you should've went on, or that job that you should've applied for, and you didn't even take out an application.

Or that degree that you were supposed to get, but you didn't even sign up for one class. Or that exercise class that you were supposed to take and you didn't even buy a pair of workout shoes or sweatpants.

Or, that business that you were going to start, that great idea that you had and you had even gone to the seminars and conferences. You did all of the research you needed to do, did the feasibility study, selected an accountant, an attorney and a banker. Everything was ready to go and at the last minute for whatever reason you backed out.

Or that date, if you were single that you should've went on; but for whatever reason decided not to go on but you asked your friend sister Susie to go in your place and she went.

And now sister Susie is married to that good-looking man that you could have been married to. And sister Susie lives in that big house that you could be living in. And sister Susie is going on those long vacations that you could be going on. And sister Susie was able to quit her job, because she now works with her good-looking husband in their own business.

Or that sport that you should've played, but you didn't even try out for the team. But brother Johnny decided to play that sport that you decided not to play. And even though he was not as good as you he is now a professional and making lots of money and is very famous. All because he tried to do the best that he could because he thought that he was worth giving his best efforts first for.

He gave his best efforts and he did everything he could to make himself the best that he could become. He worked hard to make himself better in every aspect of his game. He was always the first one to come to practice and the last one to leave.

This man made sure he ate all the rights foods; he lifted weights with the team and also did extra lifting on his own. He studied film of his opponents and learned all their weaknesses and strengths. He also had himself evaluated, to find out what he could do to make himself better.

He realized just how valuable he was and that if he would do all the things he could to uncover this value that he would be able to achieve and accomplish the goals that he had set for himself. He believed that he was worth It!!!

But it's not too late to change the way you think. It's not too late to begin to realize that you are worth it. And what I mean by "it" is that you are worth the best effort that you can put forth to make yourself the best that you can become. It doesn't matter what circumstance or situation you may find yourself in, you can still give your darn best first.

It doesn't matter how tall you may be or how short you may be, you can give your darn best first. It doesn't matter how smart you may be or how dumb you may feel you are, you can still give your darn best first. It doesn't matter how rich you may be or how poor you may be, you can still give your darn best first. It doesn't matter how old you are or how young you may be. You can still give your darn best first.

The tallest doesn't always reach the highest and the shortest doesn't always have to settle for the lowest. The smartest aren't always in the front of the class and those who feel they are the dumbest aren't always in the back of the class.

The richest doesn't always get the best and the poorest doesn't always have to end up with less. The youngest doesn't always win the race and the oldest doesn't always lose the race. But it is the one who will give his darn best first that can say at the end of the day I am the best that I can become because I gave my best first. Aren't you worth giving your best for? Aren't you? I think you are, as a matter of fact I know that you are!!

In an article by Matt Wong, on ESPN.com, updated on February 21, 2006 at the NBA All-Star game in Houston, Texas. Matt reported that "Nate Robinson and NBA player, who stands only 5'9" tall became the 2006-slam dunk champion by beating out much taller players." "Some that were 6'10". The winning dunk that Nate Robinson performed was one in which he jumped over the top of the 1986 NBA slam-dunk champion, Spud Webb, who only stands all of 5'7" tall."

What an unlikely pair to not only be able to play in what is considered to be a tall man's game. But they were able to win an event that one would think that much taller men would be more likely to win.

In his article, Mr. Wong goes on to report, "That's when Nate Rob, showing character and persistence, got himself back in the competition, walking across the court and handing Spud

Webb, his old Atlanta jersey number 4." With Web in his new duds, Robinson caught a bounce pass from the one-time dunk champ and jumped over all 5'7" of him for a spectacular jack-knife slam, finishing in a squat that he held for effect."

To make his final dunk, it took Nate Robinson 14 tries before he made the dunk in the dunk off. But it is that kind of persistence that one must have in order to be able to dig deep down inside and pullout from one's self, the kind of championship performance and effort that leaves one spent, tired, exhilarated and satisfied. Knowing that one has given his darn best!!!

The Bible records in the book of Hebrews chapter 11 that "Now faith is the substance of things hoped for, the evidence of things not seen."(Hebrews 11:1)

Nate Robertson had not yet seen the slam dunk contest victory, but he had faith that he would be able to achieve the victory. We must believe that we can do something, have that deep down faith that we can do something and then put forth the effort necessary to achieve that thing. We must become that one who will persevere, the one who will give everything that they have, the one who will not give up, that's the one that can say at the end of the day, I gave everything I had. I gave everything I could; I gave my darn best first. If you can say that then you will never be a loser and you can always feel as if you've won because you gave your darn best first. And why did you do it? Because You Are Worth it!! You Are Worth It!! You Are Worth It!!

Today, I want you to start believing that no matter whom you are, no matter what you are going through, or what you have been through. I want you to know that today, you can start changing the way you think and you can begin to put forth your best efforts in all that you do. After having done this you will begin to experience a level of satisfaction and fulfillment as never before. You will truly be able to give Your Darn Best First!!!

You Can Do IT!!

WHY?

Because You Are Worth

IT

!

Introduction

The long black limousine pulled around the corner and came to a graceful rest in front of your house. It's beautiful black glistening body shined brightly in the afternoon sun. The sun's reflection caused you to squint your eyes, as you waited expectantly for its occupants to get out. They were supposed to have arrived in the morning at around 9:30 a.m. but as with most celebrities, they are late and it was now almost 3:30 p.m. It's hot and you're sweating.

But you don't care because you would have waited for as long as it would've taken just to have someone of these celebrities' fame and status come to your house to visit you. They were your favorite stars and for a large sum of money they would come to your party sign autographs and take a few pictures with your party guest.

Slowly the driver's side door opens and the chauffeur confidently strolls around the limousine opening various doors. Out springs the three stars that you were waiting so patiently to see. The crowd went wild yelling and is screaming the celebrities' names. And who are these three celebrities?

If you wanted stars from the sports world it could be Tiger Woods, Lebron James and Peyton Manning. If you wanted stars from Hollywood maybe Brad Pitt, Denzil Washington, and George Clooney got out of the limo. If you were looking for stars from the music industry, maybe Beyonce, Justin Timberlake and Janet Jackson came to your party.

Maybe just maybe the big stars that you're waiting for were Randy Jackson, Paula Abdul and Simon Cowl. And they were coming to your house not just to sign autographs and take a few pictures; but also to conduct an American Idol program from your home. From your very own little house!!

They were going to run the full program from your home and they are going to select from a group that included you, your friends and your associates, The Next American Idol!!! And the great news is that they will be making that choice today.

It will not be necessary for you to come back next week or the following week as is the normal format with all of the other competitions. The program that you will be involved in, is a unique one-day competition and the winner will be selected right there on the spot in your home.

What's an amazing event that you are going to be a part of and what a fantastic story that you will be able to tell everyone about for the rest of your life. Your grandchildren's children will talk about this fantastic story, year after year after year. You're so excited and pleased with what you have done.

TD Jakes, Paula White and Joyce Myers could have been the celebrities if your interest was in the Christian or religious fields.

These are some of the most informative, entertaining and enlightening individuals that you could ever have come to your house. And they are there to dispense their great wisdom and knowledge to you and your guest in your home. From your very own little house and you're there to participate.

Paula could begin to tell you one of her stories about how she had been abused as a child and how she would seek refuge from her abuser by going into a closet and curling up into the fetal position shaking and crying. Or Joyce could tell you how she wanted to minister and teach people but that she did not like people. She first had to learn to like people before she was able to minister to them.

TD Jakes could launch into one of his sermons on one of the many topics that will inspire and motivate us to new levels of accomplishment and achievements.

The point is that you are very happy, because you have been able to have these very famous people to come to your home. Even though you had to wait for a long time and even though you had to pay a large sum of money. You were very pleased and you were so very excited that this trio had come to your home and that they would put on this event for you.

But what if you could have the most famous and powerful trio that will ever exist come to your house and teach you everything that you needed to know wouldn't that be great? Allow me to introduce you to them and may God bless us as we discover them together.

Chapter 1

The First Person of the Heavenly Trio: God the Father

What do I need God for anyway?
Whenever you're building anything new or refurbishing something that's not so new, let's not use the word "<u>old</u>," it is important for you to start with a good foundation. If one is going to build a new house or repair a not so new one, you must make sure that the foundation that it will sit on is solid.

The foundation, which one is going to build on must have the structural integrity to not only be able to stand-alone and withstand all the forces of nature, which will naturally come against it without breaking down. But it must also be strong enough to support the structure that we are going to put on it too. It must be solid, firm and reliable to handle difficult sitituations.

If the foundation that we build our houses upon is not strong enough to support it, our house will not have the stability that it needs and it will fall. The rains will come, and the winds will blow, everyday wear and tear will occur and eventually our house and the foundation that it is on will cave in.

But if we have the right foundation, one that is strong and powerful, and one that is able to provide the support that we need to sustain us when all the different forces began to beat against it and us trying to cause you both to cave-in under them.

The right foundation must not only take care of itself, but it must take care of you also.

" In the beginning God created the heaven and the earth (Genesis 1:1)". If God was able to create the heaven and the earth, surely he can provide the right foundation for us to build anything on, anything a building a business a career, even a life. We can build anything using God as our foundation.

The psalmist David proclaims in Psalms 55:22,

"Cast thy burden upon the Lord and he shall sustain thee:
he shall never suffer the righteous to be moved".

When the word burden is interpreted, it means our circumstances, our troubles, our cares or our problems. It does not matter what you are facing, what problems or troubles you may have, or what situation or circumstances you may be going through. If you give it to the Lord, he will sustain or take care of you. What a great promise, what a great foundation, what a great God!!! We can put anything on God He can handle it. God can take it.

I would just like to encourage any of you who are dealing with any problems or situations, which you feel you cannot overcome or it seems as if you cannot handle them and that you will never get out of whatever it is you may be facing today. I want you to know that when you put your trust in God, there is hope, because God can do everything and anything. Some times we can be facing a problem, which seems to be so great that we become depressed, discouraged and worried that we can cause ourselves to become sick.

When I was a much younger man, not saying that am old or anything now. I had to go to the dentist to have several teeth filled. The appointment was several weeks off, and as I began to think about it, I was so worried and concerned about it that I ended up losing my appetite. I literally became physically ill and would occasionally vomit with an upset stomach as the appointment date was approaching and getting nearer.

My grandmother noticed my problem and asked me what was wrong? I told her that I was afraid to go to the dentist and that I knew it was going to be painful and hurt a lot. I was so afraid of going that it was causing me to have an upset stomach and lose my appetite. She told me to just trust in God that he loves me and to believe that he would make everything all right and that everything would be fine. Then she told me something that has stuck with me for the rest of my life.

She said as a matter of fact, God loves you so much that he was willing to trade in his most valuable possession for you. It was one of a kind and the only one that he had but he was willing to trade it for you, because he loves you so much. Then she quoted these words from the Bible:

The Bible lists these words in the book of John, chapter 3, in verse 16: *"For God so loved the world, that he gave his only begotten Son, that whoso-ever believeth in him should not perish, but have everlasting life"*. My grandmother went on to say that God gave his only son in exchange for me, and she made it seem as if he had traded his only son just for me alone. We know how grandmas can tell stories and make us feel so very special and as if you are the only person in the world. She continued to say that most people when they are trading something try to get the best that you have in exchange for the worst that they have. If that doesn't work she said, then they try to increase the value a little more until finally if they have to, they will give us fair value for what they want to trade with us for.

But God did not do that; he gave the best that he had for you!! Don't you know that if God thinks that you are that special that he will protect you and take care of you while you're in the dentist chair! Don't you know that God will direct the dentist hands and protect you from any hurt or pain! She went on to say that God is so much bigger and stronger than that little old dentist that he'll make the dentist treat you right. Grandma went on to pray with me and I felt so much better that I asked her Grandma, could you please fix me something to eat. And man oh man, that food sure did taste good.

When the time came for my appointment, I was so confident that I was going to be all right that I strolled into the dentist office, sat down in the chair with a smile on my face so large that the dentist asked me what's wrong with you? What are you so happy about? The dentist said I was quite an unusual patient, and I asked him what did he mean. He said normally his patients' are happy when they leave his office, not when they come in. I told him I knew that he was going to take care of me because God and grandma had told me so. Needless to say the visit went just as grandma said it would and I was fine. Thank God for praying mothers and grandmothers, they make this cruel and mean world a safer and softer place to live! Amen! Amen! Amen! and amen!

There may be someone out there today, that may be facing something that they are so worried about that it may be causing them to become depressed and sick to the point of becoming physically ill. You may feel as if you are all alone and you don't have anyone to help or support you. You may feel as if you don't have a leg to stand on but I want you to know that you can always stand on the promises of God! He will never, never, never let you down!

In Hebrews chapter 13:6, we find these words recorded:

"so that we may boldly say, the Lord is my helper, and I will not fear what man shall do unto me".

The Merriam-Webster online dictionary defines the word help in these ways:

1: to give assistance or support to<to help the child with homework>
2a: to make more pleasant or bearable: Improve, Relieve <she took an aspirin to help her headache> 2b: archaic: Rescue, Save
3a: to be of use to: Benefit, b: to further the advancement of: Promote.

If we would just trust in God and allow his word to become real in our lives we would understand, when we need assistance or support he will be there to provide that for us just as a child receives assistance and support from its parents with his or her homework. If you have a project that you may be starting, a new job a new business or any new venture, I want you to know now that God will guide you through it. What a great foundation God is.

God will make it so that your situation will become more pleasant and more bearable. The normal ups and downs of life will not seem as difficult to deal with or as hard to handle when we allow God to direct us and we follow his instructions. If we do decide not to listen to God and we mess everything up, if we repent and change our ways he can still relieve us of our troubles and straighten out the problems we have caused because we didn't listen to him.

We can always count on God to come to our rescue, and make everything all right. We may have to pay a penalty or a price for disobeying him but if we repent and turn from our bad ways, he will never makes us pay the full price.

My parents told me that I could play football in front of my house with the children who were my own age. The surface that we played on was a brick street and sometimes we would play tackle on that brick street. I was not allowed to play with the older children, because my parents were afraid that I would get hurt if I did play with them. I told my parents that I was not afraid to play with the older kids and that I wanted to play with them. My parents told me they better not catch me out there on the street playing with the older kids. If they did, they said they were going to break my neck. I said okay and that they would never catch me out there playing with the older kids.

I was almost as big as they were and I couldn't wait to try them. I had always dominated the younger kids and I thought I was ready for the next level. I'd see the older boys out there playing and I'd start talking trash to them. I'd say; I can run as fast as you can, or I can hit as hard than you can, or I can catch as good as you can. Man, I couldn't wait to get out there and play against the older boys. I was going to beat them like they had stole something.

One day, the older kids were playing, and they needed one more player. You know who they asked don't you. That's right, they asked little old me. I remembered what my parents had told me, but since they were not around I told these older guys in my most grown-up voice, yea, sure I'll play.

Now these guys were older than me and more skilled than I was and they were beating my brains out! My nose was bleeding, I had a swollen lip and I was limping because they had knocked me down so many times on the brick street. But I couldn't let them know that they had hurt me. And I was now feeling the pain that comes with doing battle with someone that is more skilled than you are. You can give it all you have but you just don't have enough to give.

Now, I knew why my parents had told me not to play with those older boys because they were just too much more talented and stronger than I was. They also knew how to play a lot rougher than I did and they really were not concerned about my welfare or my well-being. They were only concerned about making me pay for all that trash I had talked and about winning. But I could not let them know that I was a quitter, I could not quit. They would've teased me and picked on me from that day on, I Could Not Quit!!!

My father had come home by this time, and he had been watching me play with the older boys for a little while and he could see that they were beating up on me pretty good. But my father knew that I would not quit, so my father came out and told me in the front of all of the older boys that I better get out of the game before I hurt one of them. My father said he could tell I was getting mad and was about to go off on one of them. I acted as if I didn't want to leave the game but man was I happy that my father got me out of that game!

My father gave me a way to quit without losing face in front of all the younger & older boys. My father could tell that I had suffered enough for disobeying his orders and he did not need to punish me anymore. My father wanted me to learn the lesson, but he did not want me to get killed in the process.

Sometimes our heavenly father God is like that he will allow us to do our own thing even though it's the wrong thing just so we can see that our way is not the best way. Once we have learned the lesson and have repented from the choice that we made. Then just when we think that we can't take anymore God will come in and provide a way of escape for us. What an awesome God we serve! He loves us enough to let us have free will or freedom of choice but when we mess up, God the father is there to pick us up, brush us off and let us be restored better than we were before.

From that day forward the older boys had respect for me because I did not quit and the younger boys looked at me as if I were their hero because I had played with the older boys and had not quit. This established the foundation for my reputation of being a tough player and one that would not quit. This was all made possible because my father knew what was best for me, and he acted on my behalf to provide what I needed. What a great foundation, he established for me.

We all have our heavenly father God, who is even more attentive, and concerned about us. If we would just submit ourselves to his rule and control he will provide the guidance and become the foundation we need to do anything. We can do all things with and through the power of God.

The Apostle Peter writes in first Peter chapter 5:6-7:

"Humble yourselves therefore, under the mighty hand of God, that he may exalt you in due time: casting all your cares upon him; for he careth for you".

First, Peter is telling us to humbly submit ourselves under the control or power of God and to allow God to use us in whatever way he wants to. When we do this it will permit us to be used in the best way possible. God is omniscient, which means that God knows everything. Because God knows everything, he knows how to direct us in everything that we are involved in.

We are often told that when we began any new business it is best for us to seek out those who have expertise or talents in the areas in which we are seeking to start this new business in. If we were going to start a business flipping hamburgers wouldn't it be great to have Ray Kroc, the founder of the McDonald's franchise come and mentor us and teach us everything he knew about that business.

As a matter of fact that is exactly what they do when we buy a franchise from McDonald's; they mentor us through the whole process and train us in the McDonald's way of doing business. You are sent to Hamburger University to learn all the things that it took Ray Kroc, and the other franchisees years to learn. We gain from all the trial and error they went through in the early years in developing their hamburger flipping businesses.

Someone once said that experience is the best teacher, but I want you to know I do not agree with that. I believe that second-hand experience is the best teacher, why? Because we don't have to go through all the pain, the suffering, the pitfalls, the problems and the frustrations that the one who is actually experiencing these things has to go through.

Wouldn't you rather have somebody tell you about what it's feels like to get hit in the head with a hammer then to get hit in the head with a hammer yourself? Wouldn't you rather have someone tell you what it's like to go through an earthquake, then to have to experience one yourself? Or wouldn't you rather have someone tell you about what it feels like to have open-heart surgery then to have to go through that surgery yourself? Or wouldn't you rather have someone tell you about what it's like to have had an injured back then to have to experience that injured back yourself? As I did three years ago. What a pain in the you know where that was!! I'm talking about a pain in the back, that's where, where did you think I meant? Ohh, you have a dirty, dirty, dirty mind!! Shame on you, Shame on you, shame on you.

If we had someone who could tell us how to live our lives and to be able to live our best life as effortlessly as possible? To be able to obtain the complete joy and satisfaction that comes with it, wouldn't that be great. Well, let me tell you, God is that someone who will lead us in the right direction, if we choose to submit ourselves to his leadership.

And not only will he lead us in the right direction but he will raise us up or elevate us at the right time. God will make it so that we will be appreciated for our abilities and talents. But we must make sure that we trust in him and have faith that he will do it, and then give him the glory for what he has done for us.

We must also make sure that we do the things that God wants us to do because God is just too strong for us to fight with. If God wants us to do something he can cause such hardship and pain to come into our lives that we will be sorry that we didn't obey him and do what he wanted us to do.

But if we trust God and do what he wants us to do, then God will use those same strong hands to protect us and prevent anyone from harming us. We can truly cast our burdens, our cares, and our troubles upon God, because God cares for us and he is able to prevent any hurt, harm or danger from happening to you. God cannot only support himself, but he also can support you.

That is why we need God our heavenly father, to become the starting point, the beginning to your new beginning, and the foundation for whatever it is that you are about to do. I encourage all of you today to make God the foundation of your life and to allow him to control and direct you in everything that you do. When you do you shall discover that no matter what you're trying to do, and no matter what you're going through. No matter what problems or troubles you may face, God the father is the foundation that never fails.

Chapter 2

The Second Person Of The Heavenly Trio: God The Son:

A.K.A. Jesus Christ.

W ho is this Jesus Christ Person, anyway?
Imagine if we knew someone who had unlimited resources, unlimited riches, houses and lands and he told us that we could choose any gift that we wanted. Price was no object and he would pay for it; all we had to do was make a choice. If we wanted a diamond, we could choose any diamond that we wanted to. We could choose the Cullinan I (the Great Star of Africa) the world's largest diamond, with an uncut weight of 3106 carats.

We could buy the Bugatti Type 41 Royale if we wanted to buy the most expensive automobile in the world at a price of $10 million. Imagine going to the local 7-11, in that baby. I bet we would park at the end of the parking lot or in two parking spaces. Or what about driving that bad boy to the laundromat?

We could buy the Saudi prince Bander bin Sultan's Aspen ski lodge, which lists for $135 million if we wanted to. Just think about the great parties, we could have there. We'd just have to make sure we didn't spill the tuna fish salad or the sardines on the carpet. Watch out for the chip and dip!

And there are many other expensive and high priced gifts that you could buy but you will never find a <u>gift as valuable as Jesus Christ!!</u>

The Bible explains: *"For by grace are ye saved true faith; and that not of yourself: it is the gift of God: not of works, lest any man should boast" (Ephesians 2:8,9).*

The <u>gift</u> that is being spoken about here is Jesus Christ. For if you recall in John 3:16 we are told that: *"God so loved the world that he <u>gave</u> his only begotten son, that whosoever believes in him should not perish but have everlasting life".*

God gave his only begotten son Jesus Christ as a gift to everyone who believes in him so that they would not die but have everlasting life. But why did Jesus need to be given as a gift for everyone? Why was everyone going to perish?

The Bible tells us in Romans 6:23: *"for the wages of sin is death; but the gift of God is eternal life through Jesus Christ our Lord".*

The wages or the pay or the price of sinning is death, so everyone would perish or die if they sinned, but what is sin? Sin is when you fall short of God's standards. God's standards are shown in the 10 Commandments which are listed in the book of Exodus 20:1-17. I will not list them all, but I will list some of them but I want you to look them all up in your Bible later.

The first sin I want to list is Polytheism; this is when we worship any other God but God, or we make something else our God. Now what does that mean? I used to think that it meant that we had to go out and construct a big altar, put fancy candles on it, and have a certain God or deity that we worshiped and we began to pray and bow down to that God. But all we really have to do is spend a preponderance of our time doing something. If we spend a lot of time watching television then that can be our God! If we spend a lot of time shopping, even when everything is on sale that could be our God!

There may be a special person, a football player or a basketball player or a movie star that we may bow down to and worship. Many people idolized and worshiped Elvis Presley. Many people idolize and worship Elvis as if he were a God. Elvis passed away on August 16, 1977 and still has many devoted fans that worship him to this day. There are many of his fans that believe that he is not dead but still alive and they think that they have even sited him in different places.

If you are one of Elvis's fans, as I am, and spend a lot of time pursuing Elvis or his memorabilia and if we spend more time doing that then we do worshiping God, then we are guilty of Polytheism. Now what must we do if we're spending 20% of our time on Elvis we must cut that down to about 2%, we must spend the other 98% of our time praising and worshiping God. In the book of 1st. Thessalonians 5:17 we are told to *"pray without ceasing"*, does that mean we must always be on our knees in a permanent posture of prayer? No but what it does mean is that we should pray persistently and often. "I Don't Wish to Be Cruel", but we must reduce the amount of time that we are spending with the "King Elvis", and increase the amount of time we're spending with the Real King, Jesus.

I don't want any of us to go into Elvis Presley withdrawal and start "Crying Like A Bunch Of Hound Dogs All The Time". Let's just start reading the Bible more and let's start treating Jesus like he is the "The Big Boss Man". Then we need to go out and tell people that Jesus "Wants You, Needs You And Loves You". Now I don't mean to step on anybody's "Blue Suede Shoes" or are those "Hi- Heel Sneakers", but when we need someone to tell us "That's All Right", when we're down in the dumps or "Down in the Alley" and the devil is "Trying to Get to You" and you feel like singing "A Mess of Blues", call on Jesus and he will take your blues away, he'll make it all right!!! Won't he do it! Won't he do it!! Won't he do it!!!

As stated earlier Elvis passed away on August 16, 1977, his heart stopped. Now that was over 30 years ago but we can still buy CDs, DVDs, records, movies, clothing, hats, photos and just about anything else that we can think of with Elvis's image on it. And those who are his biggest fan will pay large sums of money for these items to see his image on them. But we cannot worship God's image on anything or make something out of anything and say it is God or the image of God. Why? Because anytime we use anything that God has made to make a representation of God, it is inferior to God! If we were to make an image, or a caricature out of the most pure gold or platinum, it would still be made of inferior materials compared to God. If we do this we are guilty of committing the second sin, which is called the sin of idolatry.

Now the other sins that I'm going to talk with you about are the common ones. Swearing or making any false promises or telling lies on God. Some folks say that God has told them to do something or that their actions were directed by God and their actions really were not directed by him. They decided to do this thing themselves. They may also claim that God did an evil act and that Satan did a good one. This is known as blaspheming the name of God. Whenever you attribute to God the acts of Satan, or whenever you attribute to Satan the acts of God then you have sinned against God.

We are told: *"children obey your parents in the Lord for this is right, honor thy fathers and mothers, which is the first commandment with promise that it may be well with the and that thou may live long on the earth". (Ephesians 6:1-3)*

If we have ever disrespected our parents, talked back to them, cursed them or didn't do what they had told us to do, then we are guilty of disobeying our parents and that is a sin. We are to give them the honor and the respect that they have coming to them because they are our parents. We must first honor God so we don't have to do any sinful things if they asked us to do that.

Our mother's deserve our utmost respect just for giving birth to us. How many of us would let something that started out less than the size of a pin head, grow for nine months inside of us to become the size of a bowling ball and come out of an opening the size of a golf ball. Did I hear all the men say ouch or thank God!! Or even if your father was not around he did help you get here.

So give him respect for that, you don't have to hang out with him, respect him.

In the book of Matthew chapter 5:27 & 28, *Jesus says, "but I say unto you that whosoever looketh on a woman to lust after her hath committed adultery with her already in his heart".*

When you look upon a woman or a man, a male or female that you are not married to and you lust after them that is the sin of adultery. God only permits sexual relationships between a man and a woman who are married to one another. All other sexual unions are considered sin to God. Any sex other than marriage sex between a man and a woman who are married to each other is the sin of fornication.

Finally we are told in Exodus 20:17 "that *you shall not covet your neighbor's house, you shall not covet your neighbor's wife, nor his male servant, nor his female servant, nor his ox, nor his donkey, nor any thing that is your neighbor's".*

Covet is an interesting word that means to wish for something earnestly, with strong desire, or with excessive desire. When someone covets something, it means that they have a desire for something that is more excessive than the normal desire that one would have for something. It is like having a fixation or an obsessive desire for something or someone. Can you say the word "stalker"? We all have heard of the cases or read about the cases of celebrities being stalked by fans. How many times have we found ourselves envious or jealous of someone just because they may be able to do something better than we can. Or they may have something that's better than what we have, and we want that "something", this is the sin of covetousness.

There is another sin called gluttony that is a sin that we commit when we overindulge in anything. Eating too much food, drinking too much, watching too much television, playing too many sports, shopping too much, working out too much, etc. There is also another part to this sin of gluttony called delicacy. This sin occurs anytime we wish to have something exactly the way we want it. What do you mean brother teacher? Well what I mean my brother and sister readers, is that this person wants everything just right.

Their bathwater must be a certain temperature and only that temperature, not a degree above or beneath that temperature but that exact temperature!! Their food must be made a certain way, only put the peanut butter on one slice and only put the jelly on the other slice and then put the two slices together with the peanut butter facing down and the jelly facing up when you make them a peanut butter sandwich. I bet you thought gluttony was just a sin of overeating. As Gomer Pyle would say "Surprise, surprise, surprise."

It is not popular to talk about sin today, even in the churches. We very rarely want to hear that there is a need for us to repent of our sins and turn from our wicked ways, and turn to God. We would rather hear that all we need to do is think about the favor of God and that we are going to receive bigger and better blessings based upon how we think.

And we better not talk about Hell and the fact that it is real and it is hot and that there are no exit doors in Hell. Once we go to Hell we are there to stay. And if we go to Hell we will not be having barbecues and weenie roasts, we will be the barbecue and the weenies being roasted. That is not the way to win friends and influence people in this day and age. If we dare to discuss these subjects with friends, with associates, even with our brothers and sisters in Christ, we are often accused of discussing subjects which make people feel uncomfortable or using scare tactics to get them to believe in God. They began to avoid us like Michael Vick avoids animal rights groups!!

But what is a true friend? Is a true friend a person that tells us what we want to hear, what makes us feel good, what makes us like them and what makes us want to be their friend. Or is a true friend someone that will tell us what we need to hear, knowing that it won't make us feel good, knowing that it's unpleasant for us to hear, knowing that it could scare us and that it may cost them our friendship? Maybe this story can help us answer that question.

There was a young lady named Sister Johnson that had been waiting for a long time for just that right someone to come along. She thought she had found "Mr. Right" and she was so very happy. He said he was a "Christian", he was single, he had personality, charm, position, money, power and oh yeah, he just happened to be "fine" to. He seemed to be everything that she had been praying for. She introduced him to her two best girlfriends, Mary and Martha. About a week later Mary and Martha were out shopping and they happen to see "Mr. Right" out with another young lady. "Mr. Right" and the young lady were walking arm in arm as couples do and you could tell they were more than just friends. They were doing a lot of giggling and smiling and touching.

Mary and Martha, being the great friends that they were decided to follow "Mr. Right" and the young lady. "Mr. Right" and the young lady went to the jewelry store and "Mr. Right" preceded to purchase an ankle bracelet for the young lady. She was so elated that she kissed "Mr. Right" passionately, on the lips for almost 15 to 25 seconds, (Mary thought it was 15 seconds, Martha thought it was 25 seconds). Mary said, I've seen enough I'm leaving; Martha said I'm right beside you, I can't wait to tell Sister Johnson what we just saw. I know she'll be thankful to know the truth about this creep! Martha said I know it's going to break her heart but she'll be better off knowing the truth about him so she can dump him. Sister Johnson needs to hear this so she can move on with her life and find her real "Mr. Right"; it is what's best for her.

Mary said wait a minute, I never said I was going to tell Sister Johnson about this, you know she's going to be so hurt and she's going to be so upset, you and I both know how long she's been waiting for Mr. right, Martha. She might even get mad at us; she waited so long for her "Mr. Right" and now this. You can just see how she glows when she talks about "Mr. Right", this could cost me my friendship with her. I'm not going to say anything about this to Sister Johnson she'll find out soon enough. I'm not going to tell her the truth because I still want to be her friend and I just don't want to hurt her feelings.

The question on the table is who is Sister Johnson's true friend. Is it Mary who believes that she should keep the truth from Sister Johnson and tell her only what she wants to hear so she would not hurt her feelings and they can remain friends? Even if in the long run it causes Sister Johnson severe pain and unhappiness? Dating a man who is untrue to her. Or is it Martha? The one who is willing to tell Sister Johnson the truth even if it will hurt her feelings and could cause them to lose their friendship but in the long run it will be the best information that she could receive and allow her to make a truly informed decision about her relationship with Mr. Right.

I want to be a true friend to you today, even at the risk of making you angry or upset with me, but I am still going to tell you this one fact. There is only one way to go to Heaven and avoid going to Hell. That is who Jesus Christ is, our way to go to Heaven and to avoid going to Hell! Jesus said, *"I am the way the truth and the life: no man cometh unto the father, but by me"*. *(John 14:6)*

I do not wish to upset you nor to frighten you or anger you but I also do not wish to see you go to Hell either. So at the risk of upsetting you or making you angry, I must proceed because I love you and God loves you and he has sent me to speak with you about who Jesus Christ is. Jesus Christ is the only way for you to go to Heaven and to avoid going to Hell, why, because he is the truth of God, he is God in the flesh, he is God in human form.

As we examine John 1:1 and 1:14 which reads*: "in the beginning was the Word and the Word was with God, and the Word was God"; "And the Word was made flesh and dwelt among us, (and we beheld his glory as of the only begotten of the Father,) full of grace and truth"*.

What incredibly powerful verses that give us total and complete under-standing that before the beginning of the material universe the Word was with God. The Word was self-existing as a separate personality from God but shared deity or God ship with God The Father. He existed as the Logos, the Word of God, the utter intelligence of God, essentially in spirit form.

Who is Jesus Christ? He existed in spiritual form and then he became flesh or begun to exist in physical form or physical body. He was brought out of God and he put on a physical presence or body. He was still spirit but he now had a physical body that housed his spirit. In his physical form Jesus Christ was able to live among us and allow us to witness the power and the glory of God through him. In Jesus Christ the goodness, mercy, wisdom, truth and grace of God came alive.

The Bible states *"for we have not an high priest which cannot be touched with the feelings of our infirmities; but was in all points tempted like as we are, yet without sin"* (Hebrew 4:15). During his lifetime, Jesus Christ was exposed to the same kinds of sins that we are. He had every opportunity to tell lies but he never told one. Jesus could've stolen whatsoever he wanted and he didn't, he could have committed adultery but he didn't. He could have swore but he didn't, he could have been disrespectful and disobedience to his parents but he wasn't.

Every sin that we have been exposed to or that we could have done Jesus Christ could have done but he didn't. We all know that there are some sins which are very easy to commit and very difficult to avoid. I don't know about you but maintaining my temper and not cursing someone out has always been difficult to do. Sometimes when you haven't cursed in a while and you saved up those curse words and somebody gets you angry you just want to let them have it with those saved up curse words "in the name of Jesus."

You just go off like a machine gun burping out obscenity after obscenity. You start making up curse words, words that people have never heard before, like some new curse word language. After you've finished you can't believe you said those things. You're so embarrassed, ashamed and sorry for what you said. We don't have to be ashamed because Jesus Christ's knows all about the sins that we face because of direct first-hand knowledge and he has mercy and compassion towards us.

The Bible records these words: *"For by grace are you saved through faith and that not of yourselves it is the gift of God and not of works lest any man should boast (Ephesians 2:8-9")*.

If you recall in the previous pages there were sins that were listed. If we have committed any of those sins then we are guilty of sinning before God and as was stated before; the wages of sin is death but the gift of God is eternal life through Jesus Christ our Lord (Romans 6:23)!! If sins are committed some- one must pay the price for sinning, someone must die! But if you have made Jesus Christ Savior and Lord of your life, then he will take your place and die for you!! That's why Jesus Christ is the gift of God that allows you to have eternal life!! What a fantastic gift, what an awesome Savior, what a magnificent foundation to build your new life upon!!!

Now I know the question you are going to ask, how do I make Jesus Christ Savior and Lord of my life? Well I'm glad you asked that question because I have the answer. *Romans 10:9 & 10 reads: "That if thou shall confess with thy mouth the Lord Jesus, and shall believe in thine heart that God has raised him from the dead thou shall be saved. For with the heart man believeth unto righteousness, and with the mouth confession is made unto salvation".* When you do this you will have made Jesus Christ your Savior because he has now taken your place and he has died for your sins; and he has also become your Lord, because he will lead, direct and guide you through his word, the Bible.

Today, right now, this very moment, this very second you need to accept Jesus Christ as your Savior and your Lord! When you do you will have exchanged an eternal future in Hell, a place of torture and torment, for a brand-new eternal future in Heaven, a place full of love, joy, peace, contentment and total and complete satisfaction!!! What a fantastic trade, and all we have to do is just accept Jesus Christ as Savior and Lord of our lives. Won't you do it, won't you do it now, you have nothing to lose but an eternity in Hell and you have everything, everything, and I mean everything to gain!!!

So Right Now while it's fresh in your mind, pray this prayer with me please. Dear Lord I realize that I am a sinner and that I need Jesus Christ to trade places with me and to pay for my sins. I also need him to become my new leader and my guide so I hereby now confess Jesus Christ as my savior and my Lord. I will now begin to live for you and do what you want me to.

Now if you prayed that prayer I want you to realize that you're a brand-new creature in Christ. No longer do you have to live the way that you use to but now you can live a new life free of sin and guilt. Now what you need to do is join a good Bible believing church so you can learn about this new Savior and this new life that you are going to begin to live. And remember God doesn't need you, but he loves you and most of all he wants you to spend an eternity in heaven with him!

That's why he sent his only begotten son Jesus Christ to live a sinless life for you, so he could be a perfect sinless sacrifice for you! His son Jesus Christ was sacrificed on the cross and he died for you! He was buried in the ground three days for you but he rose from the grave on the third day for you. And now he has ascended up to heaven and he sits On the Right Hand of the Father God and he makes intercession for you!!!

What a great and wonderful God the Father And God the Son, Jesus Christ we serve, what a strong foundation to build our lives upon. Now I would like to introduce you to the final member of the heavenly trio, God the Holy Spirit. The Holy Spirit is the final part of the strong foundation we need to build or rebuild our lives upon.

I am trusting God to empower me to reveal him in all the honor and glory that he deserves. Lets us pray for each other as we proceed on this assignment together. God bless you my brothers and sisters in Christ.

Chapter 3

The Third Person Of the Heavenly Trio: God the Holy Spirit;

The Invisible Man

Why Do I Need To Have The Holy Spirit?
Imagine if we were in a fight and we wished that we had a secret weapon or a secret force to help us win the fight. I mean we were in there giving it everything that we had, fists flying, knuckle smashing against flesh, we were kicking, biting, scratching and doing about everything we could think of to win. But our opponent was doing the same thing, giving it all he had to and man was he tough! He could hit just as hard as we could, he could wrestle just as good as we could and he could take a punch just as good as we could.

If only we had an invisible friend or helper that could help us just a little bit. We're not talking about cheating, bbbbuuuuuttttt if we could just get a little help. Maybe our invisible helper could block some of those hard punches that we were getting hit with. Or maybe he could grab our opponent's hands and we would be able to have a clear shot at our opponent's chin and knock him out. Maybe our invisible friend could trip our opponent and keep him off balance just long enough for us to win! What the heck maybe our invisible helper could just pick up a board and hit our opponent in the head and just end the fight. That's ok with me, how about you? Sometimes I just want to win!!

What if we were in a debate and our competition was talking circles around us. Every time we tried to say something and developed a certain strategy he would counteract it. When we were on the offensive and were trying to press forward with our points and advance our ideas, he would shoot them down. We just could not seem to get command of our thoughts to make our points clear. And our opponent just seem to be so articulate, informative and most of all interesting and he was beating us into the ground. He was just wiping the floor with us. If only we had an invisible friend or helper who could whisper witty, interesting and exciting information to us that would help us win the debate. I'm not advocating an unfair advantage or that we should cheat, but as long as he was invisible who would know? Who would know? Who would know?

Seriously, that is what the Holy Spirit is like, an invisible helper that is able to live inside of us and is able to help us in the many ways that we need help. Jesus tells us in the 14th chapter of the book John in the 15th 16th and 17th verses: *"If ye love me, keep my commandments. And I Will Pray the Father, and he shall give you another Comforter, that he may abide with you for ever, Even the Spirit of truth; whom the world cannot receive, because it seeth him not, neither knoweth him: but ye know him; for he dwelleth with you, and shall be in you"*.

Jesus is informing us that if we love him then we will keep his commandments, but what are his commandments? Jesus in Matthew 22 tells us in versus: *"37,38,39 and 40 thou shalt love the Lord thy God with all thy heart, and with all thy soul, and with all thy mind. This is the first and great commandment. And the second is like unto it, Thou shalt love thy neighbour as thyself. On these two commandments hang all the law and the prophets"*.

We are to love the Lord God with everything that we are and everything that we have, with our complete and total being. We've got to love God with all our strength, energy and passion. We are to focus all of our human faculties totally and completely upon our efforts to love the Lord. We must give it everything that we have in showing our love for God. When we do this we are laying up treasures for ourselves in heaven to be used when we get there!

Secondly, we got to love our neighbors in the same manner, as we would want to be loved. We are to treat them, as we want to be treated, whatever we would wish to have happen to us that is what we want to have happen for our neighbors. Jesus wants to know that we are not just concerned about our own selfish desires but that we are concerned about God and others more than ourselves.

Once we keep his commandments then Jesus said he would pray the Father and he would give you another comforter even the Spirit of truth, and he will dwell in you and shall be in you. Now that we have the Spirit of truth living in us what good is it to us? If we examine John 14: 25 and 26 Jesus says: *"These things I have spoken to you while being present with you But the Comforter, which is the Holy Ghost, whom the father will send in my name, he shall teach you all things, and bring all things to your remembrance, whatsoever I have said unto you"*.

Jesus had spoken to the disciples and taught them many things while he was with them but with their natural understanding they were not able to under- stand what he was saying to them, but once the Holy Spirit came and lived inside of them they were now able to supernaturally understand what he had taught them previously. The Holy Spirit was able to energize their minds and increase their ability to understand the spiritual things of God.

Through the Holy Spirit Christians are able to function on a higher level than just the natural level or the level that our minds with their finite power function on. With the Holy Spirit we are able to understand the deeper and higher things of God and to have total understanding of those things. The Holy Spirit takes us to a higher level of consciousness, awareness and power, enabling us to go into a deeper level of power and understand that the non-Christian cannot obtain. That is why we need the Holy Spirit to take us to a higher and deeper level in our Christian lives. Now when we began to read the Word of God we have the ability to understand it because we have the Spirit of God revealing it to us. 1st. Cor. 2: 10 informs:

"But God has revealed them unto us by his Spirit: for the Spirit searches all things, yea, the deep things of God".

The Holy Spirit is the source that permits Christians to understand the revelations of God; it provides us with the ability to have contact with the mind of God. Christians are able to have intimate fellowship with God. With our secret invisible helper the Holy Spirit, Christians receive power to do the will of God. Christ tells his disciples*: "But ye shall receive power, after that the Holy Ghost is come upon you: and ye shall be witnesses unto me both in Jerusalem, and in Judea, and in Samaria, and unto the uttermost part of the earth".* (Acts 1:8). The Holy Spirit provides Christians with POWER!!! But what is power? According to the Merriam-Webster dictionary:

1. It is the ability to act or produce an effect.
2. Possession of control, authority or influence over others.
3. Physical might

The Holy Spirit provides us with power or the ability to produce something and to become effective in the things that we are involved in. To have control and authority over others and ourselves. Being able to influence our environment and make an impact upon those around us. The Holy Spirit will also allow us to have physical might and strength to accomplish the things that we start out to do. We become efficient and effective on a new and higher level that we could not obtain without the indwelling of the Holy Spirit!

This is why we need the Holy Spirit to fill us and live in us helping us to accomplish the highest and the best that God has for us. What a great helper, what a great friend but most of all what a tremendous source of power that causes us to become powerful beyond our imagination. Capable of going far beyond what we can do and achieving far more than what we ever could when we rely on just our own human abilities. What a fantastic foundation to build our lives upon. But I know what you're thinking and the question that is forming in your minds. Show us an example of someone who used this power, this Holy Spirit power, to do great and powerful things. Prove to us that someone has done this. Are all of you from Missouri or something?

In this day and age of so many different books and so many different viewpoints that tell us that we are able to empower ourselves by the way that we view our conditions and our circumstances and that all we must do is think positive thoughts and we will be able to receive anything that we want as long as we receive it or believe it in our minds. This supposed new way of thinking tells us that the way we think will cause us to draw or attract positive or negative things in our lives. In other words it is not God as Father, Son and Holy Spirit that should be in control of our lives and destiny but it's how we think that will determine what we are and what we accomplish.

Then there are religious philosophies that proclaim that we are God and that there is no difference between God and us. That God is us and we are God. But I would like to introduce you to the most powerful man that ever walked the face of the earth, one who used this power, introducing the Lord Jesus Christ!!!

Chapter 4

Holy Spirit Power

The Power to Pass Every Test.

As we examine the fourth chapter of the book of Matthew starting with verse one and concluding in the 4th verse we find these words recorded as a testimony and conclusive proof of the power of the Holy Spirit. Verse 1 reads:

"Then was Jesus led up of the Spirit into the wilderness to be tempted of the devil". What an interesting verse, it states that the Spirit led Jesus into the wilderness to be tempted or tested of the devil. One would think that the Spirit would be leading Jesus away from the temptation or the test, keeping him safe and protecting him from the devil. We often are told that when we become a Christian we would be protected from any hurt, harm or danger so why is the Holy Spirit leading Jesus into harms way?

Maybe I can use a athletic analogy to explain my point. When we are training to run a race we must first of all face the fact that we are going to have to run to participate in the race and hopefully win. If we do not run in the race and everyone else is running chances are we are not going to win the race. If Jesus' opponent is the devil then Jesus is going to have to face him to win. As soon as the Holy Spirit came in and indwelled Jesus, he was ready to get it on with the devil. He didn't waste any time and he went right to the place that he knew he would find the devil, in the wilderness. And we should learn a couple of lessons from this, first we should understand that when we become Christians the Holy Spirit is not going to lead us away from the battle but he will lead us into the midst of the battle. But please note and be aware of the fact that the Holy Spirit is leading, he's out in front not beside or behind us.

The Holy Spirit is not afraid of fighting and we, as Christians should not be either. We need to understand that once we line up on the Lord Jesus Christ's side, we automatically become the enemy of the devil and he's looking for a fight. So you better get ready to do some fighting. Secondly, when we go into the wilderness we better expect to find some bad things, some demonic thing, and some devilish things. But don't be afraid because if you are a Spirit filled believer being led by the Holy Spirit you have the greatest fighter that there is leading you in the battle. As these verses will show he fights to win.

Verse 2, 3 & 4 continues: "And when he had fasted 40 days and 40 nights, he was afterward an hungered. And when the tempter came to him he said, if thou be the Son of God, command that these stones be made bread. But he answered and said, it is written Man shall not live by bread alone, but by every word that proceedeth out of the mouth of God".

After fasting for those 40 days and 40 nights he was hungry and one can understand that. When we think about doing without food we think that we've done something if we have breakfast, skip the snack and just have lunch. Some of us more dedicated fasters may go for three or four days and we realize the will power that it takes to do that. So we can imagine how hungry Jesus must have been when the tempter came to him. And the devil knew exactly what to attack Jesus with; he knew he had been fasting and that he should be hungry. The devil does not fight fair and he looks for any advantages.

The devil can attack us at our weakest point and during our weakest moments. Under our own natural strength we would not be able to resist this attack but being empowered by the Holy Spirit Jesus was strengthened and was able to resist the first temptation, and that same power is available to us through the Holy Spirit!! Jesus Christ must have been extremely weak and needed and wanted to eat but he was able to put aside his wants and needs and tell the devil what the written Word of God said. But what did Jesus mean when he said man does not live by bread alone but by every word that precedents out of the mouth of God?

We are told in John 6:63: It *is the Spirit that quickeneth, the flesh profiteth nothing: the words that I speak unto you they are spirits and they are life.* This verse lets us know that the spirit is quickened or made alive or is given life by the word of God. The word energizes the spirit and allows it to have the power that it needs to function on a higher level and in a higher dimension. When Jesus says man lives by every word that proceeds out of the mouth of God he means that the word is food for the Spirit. When a Spirit filled Christian reads the word of God he receives power and nourishment just as if he were being fed a satisfying full course dinner. When Jesus quoted this verse his Spirit was energized with supernatural power like an empty battery being recharged to its full capacity. Jesus was like a runner who had received his second wind and he had renewed strength and power to fight the devil.

But something also happened to the flesh or the body of the Spirit filled believer, the verse says the flesh profiteth or benefits nothing (Jn. 6:63), or the flesh gets nothing from the Word of God. Our flesh receives no nourishment or fuel to live from the word of God. When we don't give our flesh any fuel to live our flesh dies. Now what do you mean brother teacher? If our flesh is not nourished or does not receive any food then We Will Die too! That's can't be a good thing! Explain this thing to us; please make it plain so that we can understand because we do not want to Die Just Because We Read the Word of God!!! We like our flesh we just do not like some of the things that it does some time. But we don't want to kill it; we just want to have more control over it. Because sometimes after we have eaten that whole pack of cookies, and we only were going to open up the pack and eat just one or at the most five, or the times when we find ourselves eating that fourth plate of food at the buffet when were only were going to have the salad; we would like to have more control of our flesh and its appetites.

Our bodies do not die literally but what happens is that the desires of the flesh or the fleshly appetites are starved to death because the word of God is to deep for the natural man, the worldly man or the carnal man to be able to get anything out of it. His fleshly appetites will no longer rule the carnal or worldly man and it will now be easier for him to be controlled by the Holy Spirit. The next chapter should help us understand this more clearly.

Chapter 5

Spiritual Revelation for Deeper Understanding And Power

In First Corinthians Chapter 2:9-15 we find these words that should offer some clarity and understanding in how to obtain Spiritual control over our lives and our bodies with their fleshly and worldly appetites.

"But as it is written, Eyes have not seen, nor ears heard, neither have entered into the heart of man, those things which God hath prepared for them that love him. But God has revealed them unto us by his Spirit: for the Spirit searches all things, yea, the deep things of God. For what man knoweth the things of a man, save the spirit of man which is in him? even so the things of God knoweth no man, but the Spirit of God. Now we have received, not the spirit of the world, but the Spirit which is of God; that we might know the things that are freely given to us of God. Which things also we speak, not in the words which man's wisdom teacheth, but which the Holy Ghost teaches; comparing spiritual things with spiritual. But the natural man receiveth not the things of the Spirit of God: for they are foolishness unto him: neither can he know them, because they are spiritually discerned. But he that is

spiritual judgeth all things, yet he himself is judged of no man."(1ˢᵗ Corinthians 2:9-15)

The eyes, ears, the heart or being of the natural man can not understand the deeper things of God because the natural man does not have the Spirit of God which reveals these things to him. He is similar to a person that has a radio and he's trying to download information from the Internet. His radio is not equipped to receive the downloads because it is just too primitive and antiquated to receive those downloads. The Internet functions on a higher level than the radio and the radio cannot receive or get anything from the Internet. That is why the Word of God is foolishness to the natural man, because he cannot receive the download from God. He does not have the proper equipment to receive the download and use the word of God to control his flesh. The only weapon that the natural man has to control himself is the spirit of man, which is willpower or the wisdom and knowledge of the world.

Now what wisdom and knowledge does the world use to control the natural or carnal man. Well I'm glad you asked that question because I think I know the answer. All the wisdom and knowledge that the world uses comes from the same spirit of man that the problems which they are trying to solve comes from. Whatever therapies or treatments are being employed to address the problem comes from the minds of men. Because the problem and the solution are on the same level, one is no more powerful or stronger than the other. Because one is no stronger than the other, the results of the treatment normally are determined by the desire or willpower of the person who is being treated to get better. If the person is strong willed and has a strong desire to get well then chances are the treatment will work. But if the person does not have a strong will chances are the treatment will fail. That is why every good practitioner will always tell us that every treatment outcome depends on how badly we wish to get well or our willpower. What we need is to have something or someone more powerful and stronger then the problem that we are facing.

This is why you find so many individuals who will go into a rehabilitation program for 28 days, 45 days or however long the program may be and will come out of rehab and some of them will be riding home from rehab smoking a joint or smoking some crack or grabbing a drink on the way home from the rehab center. When the stimuli or the substance that they were trying to quit was not around then they could stop using. Why because they had enough will power to abstain from the substance when it was not in their presence. But once they were exposed to the substance again they didn't have enough willpower to abstain and they began to use the substance again.

But can I go deeper? No problem, thank you. The problem that they went to rehab for and the solution were on the same level. But when you go to a deeper, stronger more powerful source for the solution than the solution can handle the problem. When you have that all mighty powerful Holy Spirit of God living in you, being nourished by the Word of God. Now we have a solution that is more powerful than the problem!!! Now we have a great opportunity not for rehabilitation but for transformation.

The Bible says, *"be not conformed to this world: but be ye transformed by the renewing of your mind that you may prove what is that good and acceptable and perfect will of God"* (Romans 12:2). Rehab programs are designed to change your behavior, but the Holy Spirit and the Word of God is designed to change all of you!! How you behave, how you think, how you live, your whole being, your whole mind, your whole life! Can I go deeper? That is why Jesus Christ could say to the devil; man does not live by bread alone but by every word that proceedeth out of the mouth of God. Even when Jesus had a real need for food and a real need to eat to stay alive when confronted and tempted by the devil. Jesus received supernatural power from the Holy Spirit and the Word of God to be able to resist the temptation!! And this was not an acquired habit like smoking or snorting crack or marijuana, or drinking, etc., this was a real need that Jesus had to eat or he would die. If you don't eat you do not live but Jesus was able to resist the devil and turndown the temptation of making the stone into bread.

The natural or the carnal man would say that Jesus Christ was a fool for not turning the stone into bread and eating to satisfy his hunger. But Jesus was on a greater mission from God to satisfy God's will and not his own. Too often we are told in today's church messages that God is here to do our will and that we need to make demands upon God for all our wants and desires. But when we examine this example by Jesus, when he was willing to give up a function that was vital in keeping him alive in order to show his desire and willingness to do God's will; we must conclude that we can do no less. We should be willing at all costs to do God's will and realize that God will take care of us.

Can I go deeper? Thank you. The carnal man would ask why should I do the will of God at the expense of doing my own will? Don't I deserve to be happy? Don't I deserve to be able to satisfy myself? Don't I deserve to at least eat? I deserve that don't I? The carnal man has a worldview and he is unable to understand anything else that is above that level. The Bible explains: *"For we wrestle not against flesh and blood, but against principalities, against powers, against the rulers of the darkness of this world, against spiritual wickedness in high places."*

The fight is not against a physical opponent but a spiritual one and the battle is just not over eating, it is over whom we are going to serve or obey. The fight is over who is going to control our minds.

The devil wants us to serve him and he will appear at our darkness and lowest moment bringing what we really think we need or think we want to see if he is able to tempt us. The devil will also try to have us do something that he suggests in an attempt to have us trust in him and not trust in God. He wanted Jesus to fulfill his own needs and not trust in God to feed him. But Jesus was depending upon God to be his source. He knew if he were to feed himself by turning the stone into bread then God would not be his source and he would have been disobedient to God. The devil would have been successful in controlling his mind and causing him to do what he wanted him to do.

What has the devil been tempting you with? How has he been tempting you to rely upon yourselves and not upon God? Has he been telling you that it's okay to play the lottery? We know if we don't play we can't win those millions of dollars. Often times many of the people who have won don't have very much money left 5 or 10 years after they have won. Games of chance or gambling should not be used, as the source to satisfy our needs for money God should be the source.

What about that friend that you have on the side? Our wife or our husband doesn't know about him or her and as long as we take care of business at home what's the harm in having a little outside fun? Adultery is a sin and will only bring us much more grief then the little pleasure that we shall receive in the end. So what if we are spending hour after hour watching television or playing video games on our computers, it's our time, we can use it as we want to can't we? What about all the time we are spending at the gym or the club working out three or four hours a day? What's the harm in using our time to improve our health and our bodies?

The devil wants to get our attention focused on anything else but God, and he wants us to look upon any other source but God to fill our needs and wants. When this occurs it is not long before our attention becomes focused on the devil. We must always remember that there is a battle going on in the high places between God and the devil and what they're fighting over is the control of our minds.

To serve the devil all we need to do is live and the things in this world are designed to promote the devil's agenda. Watch television and we will see some of the most hedonistic and devilish things known to man. There is a barrage of sex, violence, disrespect and disregard for human life. Children are encouraged to be disrespectful to parents and parents are portrayed as weak and permissive with no idea how to raise their children and providing any discipline to their children is just out of the question.

The Internet is a very useful tool that can provide much information and can be a source of data and entertainment but if used improperly it can bring many disgusting and revolting images into our homes to be viewed by our family members and children. There are also many sites that show pornographic materials and sites that have many pedophiles and predators waiting to pounce on unsuspecting children. It takes very little effort to serve the devil, the world seems to be full of his pitfalls and booby-traps.

It takes some effort on our part to serve God in winning this battle. There is an old saying, "anything worth wanting is worth waiting for." But I would like to say, "anything worth wanting is worth working for." We must repent and turn away from our worldly ways, accept Jesus Christ as Lord and Savior of our lives, talk with God in prayer, read the Word of God to strengthen our spirits and witness to others to promote the kingdom of God. But the effort is worth it, because the reward is to be able to go to heaven and to lead others there also. We are laying a foundation for a successful life while we are on this earth and after when we leave it. I think it's worth the effort to be able to go to our heavenly home and live an eternity with God the father God the son and God the Holy Spirit!!

Often times in our lives we face many challenges and we must decide if we are going to let these events rule and ruin our lives or are we going to roll up our sleeves, square our shoulders, lock our jaws, bull our necks, plant our feet and get ready to make a stance against all of the attacks and challenges of the devil. Are the things that we want to achieve and accomplish for the Lord worth fighting for? Are the things that we want to achieve and accomplish for the Lord worth our giving our best efforts and giving it everything that we have? To be able to hang in there if necessary until the end, to be able to persevere for as long as it takes for the glory and honor of the God we serve.

We have to put one very important thought in our minds and that is this, that whenever we say that we are Christians the world is going to begin to look at us as being a representative of Jesus Christ. Everything we do will be scrutinized and examined to the most miniscule degree to find any flaws; faults or cracks in our armor. The world will be hoping that we fail to live up to the standards of God and the devil will be doing everything he can to make that happen. The devil will bring all of the forces of hell and his legions of demonic spirits against us. He and they are formidable foes make no mistake about it.

In First John these words are provided to encourage us in our battle: *"Ye are of God, little children, and have overcome them: because greater is he that is in you, than he that is in the world."(1st. John 4:4)*. John was speaking about all of the spirits that are in the world and the source of their origin, which is the Antichrist. John was letting us know that we have the greatest spirit of all which is the Holy Spirit living inside of us, and the Holy Spirit is greater than the Antichrist and any of the other spirits that are in the world. Because we have the greatest spirit living inside of us no matter what spirit we have to contend with we can overcome it.

If we are facing a spirit of doubt, the Holy Spirit in us is greater than that spirit of doubt and we can overcome it. If we us facing a spirit of fear the Holy Spirit that is in us is greater than that spirit of fear and we can overcome it. If we are facing a spirit of inferiority the Holy Spirit that is in us is greater than that spirit of inferiority and we can overcome it. If we are facing a spirit of poverty the Holy Spirit inside of us is greater than that spirit of poverty and we can overcome it. If we are facing a spirit of depression the Holy Spirit inside of us is greater than that spirit of depression and we can overcome it. If we are vexed or made sick by a spirit of grief such as David was, (2nd Sam 12: 10) the Holy Spirit inside of us is greater than the spirit of grief and we can overcome it. We can overcome any spirit that comes against us because the spirit inside of us is greater !!

And I know the question that is on your mind; you're asking how do I know we can overcome any spirit that comes against us? I know because I have had to use my faith and my trust in God the father God the son and God the Holy Spirit and the Word of God to empower me to fight the battle of my life against many of the spirits mentioned in the sentences above. With this foundation I was able to regain my spiritual, mental and physical health on a level that I had not obtained before!!

I'm not saying that I can run as fast or jump as high as when I was 18, nor am I about to play football again. But physically I feel as good as I've ever felt and I can still run, jump and lift weights, something that doctors told me that I could not do.

I feel so good again at 55 years old I feel like I have been renewed, I feel as if I have been reborn,

I Feel As If I Have Come Alive at 55!!!!!!!!Many folks seem to believe that when you reach the magic double nickel that it's time to break out the rocking chair and then call the undertaker. But I'm here to tell you that at 55 you're not dead you're alive and the best is ahead of you!! And I will show you how you too can come alive. If you will permit me I would like to tell you my story. May God bless us as we unfold these truths together and may you be encouraged and empowered in your own personal battles with the devil!

ARE YOU READY TO COME ALIVE AT 55
Dr. M. D. Brown, 1st.

Chapter 6

Just Another Ordinary Day

The mellow sound of the singer's voice filled the cabin of the luxury SUV. The vehicles six televisions, DVD player, VCR and rear stereo system lay dormant as the front CD was individually presenting a performance that would make any concert hall audio system turn green with envy. The crooner's silky and velvety voice made each song sound as if he was born to sing it.

It did not matter to me that he was singing gangster rap, it did not matter to me that some of the lyrics were rather explicit, I just liked his voice and I was going to listen to it and who was going to stop me? Who was I hurting? What damage or harm was I doing to anyone? I only played it when I was alone.

After all wasn't I a preacher, a former pastor and founder of a Church, a radio host and an entrepreneur, that owned several businesses and was now Administor of an organization which helped people reach their full potential? I could do what I wanted to, I was a darn full-grown man. What was the harm in listening to a little good music? Didn't I try to do the right things? I was kind of proud of the way that I've been living my life, staying out of trouble and taking care of my family and taking care of myself.

That morning, like most of them I got up at about 5:30 a.m. read my Bible for about an hour and worked in my business for about an hour. After that I got on the treadmill and put in 5 miles. Twice a week I would lift weights instead of running.

I could bench press over 300 pounds and at age 50 that wasn't too shabby. Yes indeed, I was very much pleased, you could say proud of myself.

How many of you know that the Bible says: *"Pride goeth before destruction and an haughty spirit before a fall". (Proverbs 16: 10)* Sometimes we just don't realize how arrogant and prideful we have become just because we feel that we may not be doing some of the big sins like adultery, stealing, drinking, drug addiction etc. but pride and self-righteousness are also sins. A proud look is an abomination to God and he hates it. (Proverbs 6: 16-17) The way I was acting God could not have been too happy with me but at that point I was more concerned about pleasing myself then I was about pleasing God.

Back in the SUV, as the music began to sound better and better as the singer went through his runs of cool rhymes and riffs, I decided to grab a cold bottle of water from the vehicle's refrigerator. As I sipped on the drink I couldn't help but feel satisfied with myself for deciding to design and equip this vehicle the way I had.

Besides the aforementioned amenities the vehicle also had a custom dashboard, custom steering wheel, custom burl wood treatment, grill guard, rear guards, vent shades, heated power seats, custom tires and rims, On Star telephone system and also a heating unit to keep food warm. What a nice vehicle, what a great mode of transportation, what an ego trip.

As I was proceeding to my destination, my left hand gently caressing the custom made steering wheel as I maneuvered the SUV down the street. My right hand brushed across the Armani trousers that I was wearing. I quickly glance over at the suit coat that I had draped over the passenger's front seat to ensure that it was still in place, wrinkle free. Everything looked just right.

But how many of us know that when everything seems to be going just right, when everything seems to be just perfect, when everything seems too good to be true that's when we better look out. That's when we better duck!

This was just like any other ordinary day in my life and you know it's really strange how ordinary days and unusual days often times start out the same. We get up and prepare for our unusual day just like any other ordinary day. Everything proceeds as usual, everything seems to be going right and then the tragedy happens, the accident occurs, the catastrophe strikes and hits us like a ton of bricks.

Sometimes we are never the same after a tragedy. Often times we began to feel sorry for ourselves and wonder why God is allowing this to happen to us; and we feel as if he is being cruel or unfair to us. This can cause us to have the wrong attitude toward God and look upon the tragedy in the wrong way. We may feel that we are not as bad as someone else and that they would be more deserving of this type of punishment then we are. We may think something like God, why don't you do this to my brother or my sister, they are real bad.

But if we have the right attitude and trust that God is sovereign and in control of everything and let the tragedy have the desired effect, just like Job, the Lord will bless our latter end more than our beginning (Job 42:12). In other words God may use the tragedy to correct or chasten us; we will suffer loss and have to endure great pain, but it won't be permanent. We will learn our lessons and repent from our wicked ways and by his grace God will restore us with more than we ever had before.

My daughter Camille had a situation just like that this past summer. After being in her field for almost 8 years she was let go from her job through no fault of her own. Finding herself unemployed she could've taken the attitude that God was punishing her for no reason at all and that he was being unjust toward her. She could have gotten mad at God and became withdrawn and depressed and just given up, continuing to dwell on the negative situation she was experiencing.

Knowing that God is always fair and just, instead of blaming him for her situation she began to examine herself and look for areas that she needed to correct in her life. As she was doing this she discovered some areas that she felt that she could improve upon and that would please God. She used the time to become closer to God, she began to pray and read her Bible more. Camille had not been as close to God as she had wanted to be for almost 17 years. It was during that time that she had an illness that had rendered her unable to walk or talk and she even had to have a tracheotomy to assist her in breathing. She was placed in a nursing care facility to help her recover from her illness.

While she was unemployed she began putting in applications for new jobs. She was hoping to get just another job similar to the one she had before. A good friend told her about a position that was opening up and Camille applied for the position. She interviewed for the position and was impressive but she did not have as much education or experience as some of the other candidates. She was called back for a second interview and she was just overjoyed and grateful to God that she was called back for a second interview. As happy as she was you would have thought she had gotten the position!

The company's policy for new hires in positions such as this was to have the perspective position candidate have a third interview with the executive director of the company before they were hired. On the second interview the interviewer that was interviewing Camille was so impressed with her that he hired her on the spot. He told her that he knew the executive director would like her and that he was not going to let her get away. He told her that she did not have as much education or experience as some of the others but that she had sold herself so well that they would train her to be able to do the other duties that the position required. Talk about the favor of God! Isn't God good!

How many of you know that God is able to do exceedingly abundantly above all that we ask or think according to the power that worketh in us (Ephesians 3: 20). Camille was just looking for a job; anything to put some money in her pocket and to pay the bills but God gave her a position. Cam had some power that was working in her. She was one of the top speakers in the nation in individual interpretation while in high school, finishing third in the nation as a junior and senior. She was trained to speak and knew how to present herself. Her friend told her about the opening up but she had to fill it.

And fill the position she did, what a great testimony that showed the fantastic and awesome power of God. He can do anything, there is nothing that God cannot do but fail. Camille could have been discouraged because she didn't have as many degrees or experience that the other candidates had but she had a foundation of faith, dependent upon God and she knew that he would make a way for her. She also maintained an attitude of praise, thanking him and being glad and grateful for everything that God was doing for her.

Psalms 22: 3 informs *"But thou art holy, O thou that inhabitest the praises of Israel"*. God lives in the praises that we send up to him. He loves praise. When we show God that we will praise him even when the situation doesn't justify that we have anything to praise him for, just watch God show out in our lives. Camille praised God every step along the way of her interview process and he just kept on doing more and more for her. It wasn't her fault that she found herself unemployed but you know sometimes in our lives we're going to have trials, tribulations and unfortunate events to overcome but if we have faith in God he will bring us through. If she hadn't been unemployed from her other job than she would not have found the great new position she has now.

But God has a way of leveling the playing field; God has a way of making everything work out if we will just trust in him he will bring us through! Won't He Do It, Won't He Do It, Won't He Do It!!!

And What He Has Done for Her He Will Do for You!!!

I bet you're wondering what the position is that Camille now has aren't you? If you give me $500.00 I'll tell you. But seriously Camille is now employed in the position of the Director of Admissions and Marketing, at <u>**A NURSING CARE FACILITY!!**</u> Isn't God Great!!

God can take your misery and turn it into a ministry; God can take your mess and turn it into a message. I don't know whom I'm talking to but there's somebody out there today who is going through pure D. Hell in your life. You feel as if there is no way out, you believe that there is no way that you are going to make it and that all of the pressures and the pain and the depression is going to cause you to lose your mind. But I want you to know today that if you will just hang in there, today if you would just hold on, today if you will hold out, today if you will continue to trust and believe in God I know God will pull you through!!! Do it today! Do it today!

This shows that no matter what age you are these principles of God will work for you. If you keep your faith in God alive he will give you the desires of your heart. Why don't you try them and encourage whomever you know to try them too. They will not be sorry they did. But now let's go back to the SUV.

Chapter 7

Every Child Should Have Good Parents: Even Grown-Up Ones

Back in the SUV, I begin thinking about how nice it was to be able to run my own businesses and I was also in the process of activating M.D.B.1, a ministry that I was very excited about. I knew this ministry was much needed and I had a great passion and desire to get it started. How blessed and smart I was to be able to do the things that I was doing. If it weren't for the fact that I might wrinkle my shirtsleeve I would have patted myself on the back.

My favorite saying when someone would ask me how are you doing I would say, I feel so good that I swear I have died and gone to heaven. Man, was I clean, looking good and feeling great. Man, what a beautiful day. What was today's date anyway? Let me check my Rolex, October 31, 2003!!

<u>Halloween</u> !!!

I had agreed to speak at a funeral and I was almost there, only about six more minutes from my destination. I was now in the center lane on a four-lane street. The car in front of me had stopped to make a left hand turn & I proceeded to come to a complete stop behind him. I'd been stopped for approximately five seconds when all of a sudden I felt this tremendous collision and impact from behind. It was as if I had been smacked directly in my lower back by a board, a 2 x 4 or an old wooden paddle; like the kind that teachers used to use to give you a spanking with. What's going on? What just happened?

"Chasten thy son while there is hope, and let not thy soul spare for his crying"(Proverbs 19: 18). "And ye have forgotten the exhortation which speaketh unto you as unto children, My son, depise not thou the chastening of the Lord, nor faint when thou art rebuked of him: For whom the Lord loveth he chasteneth, and scourgeth every son whom he receiveth"(Hebrews 12: 5, 6) These verses are letting us know about a very important subject that has been a source of great controversy and that is, does God allow or permit bad things to happen in our lives? When we read these verses we are being instructed to chasten or correct our children before they reach a point where they cannot be corrected and where we will not be able to reach them.

When little Johnny is five or ten years old you can talk things over with him and make him understand. But when little Johnny turns into big John at about 16 or 17 years of age now it's a little tougher to give John a talking to. Heck at that age it's difficult to provide any kind of discipline to big John. At that age he's probably towering above you and could overpower you! I can hear you now, watch out here comes big John and he's got a belt! Everybody run, big John is going to get you.

My mother did not care how old or big you were, she would tell you if you don't listen to what I say I'm going to hit you with my shoe. She'd take her shoe off and throw it at you from anywhere in the house. You start mouthing off and complaining about something before you were finished talking you had a M.F.O. (Mother's Flying Object) hitting you in your head!! Man did those high heels hurt. And mom would tell you that if you didn't like getting hit with the shoe then you better do what she said. Mom also let all of us kids know that if we got to bad she could always trade a pair of shoes in for a baseball bat.

If we provide direction and correction to our children early on in life and not give in because they began to protest or cry, our children will know how to behave when they get older. I have witnessed many parents who have given in to their children while disciplining them simply because the child did not want to participate in the discipline because the discipline was unpleasant. You know what I say about that, DUH!!!! None of us wish to get disciplined or go through anything that is unpleasant however if we don't have to face something unpleasant we may never change our behavior even for our own benefit.

If we tell a child not to touch the stove and he ignores us and touches the stove anyway and he gets a slight sensation of being burned, the unpleasant- ness that he experiences causes him to understand that we were trying to prevent him from being burned. He should then learn the lesson of not touching the stove because he will get burned. It is unfortunate that we must sometimes experience unpleasantness in order for us to learn a lesson. Too bad we don't have the discipline to listen to and do what's right all the time.

Self-discipline in a child can only be achieved when the parent helps him to develop discipline. Without a parent guiding the child and making sure that the child has certain standards to abide by and making sure the child adheres to those standards; the child does not have much of a chance of developing any discipline whatsoever.

That is one of the reasons why we have the problem of childhood obesity. Parents give in to their children before the children can learn the self-discipline of eating the right types and the right amount of foods. Then as the children get older they continue on this course of eating unhealthy foods that they now have acquired a taste for.

The parents also give in to their children by giving the children food to eat to keep them quiet. Even if the child is not hungry the parent will use the food as a pacifier, just something to keep the child occupied and out of their hair. Instead of putting in real parenting time and teaching the child how to learn to sit quietly they stuff a piece of meat in their mouths and go on about their business. Come on young parents raise your children by biblical standards. Join a Bible believing church, read the Bible and Counsel with your pastor. Counsel with some of the older parents and couples who have raised children they'll be happy to assist you. But now back to the SUV.

The verse also tells us that as sons of father God, we have made the choice to do his will, we should not become angry or hate God when he decides to discipline us. We should accept whatever God chooses for us because we have turned our will over to him and have put our faith in him to do whatever it is that he feels is best for us. We trust him to be fair and just in controlling our lives and whatever he decides to do will be beneficial to us in the end.

We have been influenced to believe that if a person is a bad person and has not been living a godly life that they will not receive any good things in life. We think that this is revealed & expressed by the amount of things that they have and the state of health that they are in. We think that these people will be plagued with poverty and bad health. Living a life filled with sickness and want. They will be in a state of what we normally called being "down and out".

But there are many people that live ungodly lives and have never so much as cast a shadow near a church door or whose fingers have never caressed the Holy Word of God. They have all the signs of success and seem to exhibit great health. They have the money, the homes, the prestige and popularity that go along with what we would call the image of "the good life." And these people will not acknowledge God and do not have a desire to know him. As a matter of fact they will attribute all their successes to themselves. These people are in a different kind of state, they are in the state of what we will classify as being "up and out". They have stuff and they believe that they are the ones who got that stuff, on their own, with no help from anybody else, especially not God.

Sometimes when we think that we are doing just great and that there is nothing that we can do to improve upon our lives or our relationship with God.

That's when we may be the farthest away from him. We often equate having things, houses, cars, lands, business successes, multiple streams of income, health and just living the good life in general as being evidence that we are doing the will of God and are receiving the blessings of God. We have been acknowledging God and praising him for what he has done for us, But we have become self-righteous and important and very very arrogant because of the blessings of God and the benefits that we are receiving from our relationship with him.

Sometimes if we're not careful we can exploit or use our relationship with God. As a matter of fact we may have little rituals that we go through just to show that God is blessing us. You know those sayings we use, how are you doing today? Oh I am blessed by the best, amen. We have Christian ring tones on our telephone. We know just what to say and we know just what to ask. We just don't really mean it. We learn how to speak "Christianize", the Christian slang that lets us sound real religious but we have no real relationship with Christ. We are playing around with our walk with God! But God wants us to take our walk with him seriously or he will allow serious things to happen to us to let us know how serious he is. This accident was a serious thing.

Now Back to the SUV!

Chapter 8

Big Surprises Come in Small Packages

I took a moment to get myself together and gather my thoughts. Don't panic, stay calm, don't get emotional, relax, assess the situation, take inventory of what just happened and take the appropriate action. You're an administrator, a former pastor, a problem solver, you put out fires, and you're trained to be calm under fire. I can feel the adrenaline kicking in now, take a deep breath and let's go. Remember your four P's, professional, poised, polished, powerful.

I looked in my rearview mirror and I could just barely see the top of the little car that had struck me from behind. Okay, I've been in a car wreck; I've been rear ended, how do I feel? A little confused, my body feels okay but my back is hurting. I can't believe this has happened to me especially on the way to a funeral. I'm starting to get a little angry, stop that right now because that will not help; Come on let's get it together Now. Time to call 911. Call my wife.

After the calls I got out of the SUV and went to the back of the SUV to look at the damage to it and the vehicle that had caused the damage. The first thing that I noticed was that this was a very small compact car. My great big SUV had very little damage to it, (found out later only $1200) and it was no more than a little dent to the bumper. It was reported to be one of the safest vehicles on the road and it seemed to have lived up to its reputation. I was very pleased that I had selected this SUV. Only the bumper appeared to be slightly damaged but I did have that little pain in my back.

I also noticed that the front end of the car that had hit me was smashed in all the way back almost to passengers compartment. It looked like an accordion! I was thinking that I would be fine after looking at the scene. The man who had been driving the car that hit me had come out and asked me was I okay and said that he and his passengers were okay. I explained to him that I had some pain in my back but that I knew I would be okay. It was only a little pain but I was going to go back to my SUV and sit down and wait for the police to come. As I walked back to my SUV I kept thinking about how little that car was.

"Take us the foxes, the Little foxes, that's spoil the vines: for our vines have tender grapes."(Songs of Solomon 2:15)

As a pastor and a minister I have seen many situations that started out small and then just escalated into very large problems. I witnessed married couples that seemed to be the perfect couple last year, very happy and extremely in love with each other, one partner hurt the other partner's feelings and now they're heading for divorce court. Just because he forgot to pick her up from work one day. Or she spent a little more money than she should have. I've visited people in jail who have gotten into a fight and ended up killing the other person because they believed that the person had been disrespectful because they had been staring at them too long. "What are you looking at?"

I have seen people with very small spots on their arm that have turned into cancer and spread throughout their whole bodies and caused their death. I have heard of people who said they felt just a little dizzy but later on it was found that they had cancer of the brain and died. I've seen churches breakup and split because they could not decide what colors to wear for men or women's day.

It's those little foxes that spoil the vine; it's those little things that can cause big problems. I'm sure that many of you know of someone or some event that started out so very small but turned into something so very large. We never would have believed that such a small thing could have snowballed and caused such a big problem. Such little things can sometimes change the outcome of so many situations in such a big way.

My mother, God rest her soul, really believed in herbal remedies and cures. One time she told me about this treatment that I could use to shrink bumps. She told me that if I would make a paste out of oatmeal and put it on bumps that it would shrink the bumps and make them go away. I tried it on a bump that I had on my face and the oatmeal paste completely shrunk the bump in one-day. I was very excited, I was very happy and I thanked my mother for her advice by taking her to dinner. We had a great time because I really enjoyed talking to my mother very much. She was a great lady and I really loved her. Mom had so much knowledge and wisdom and such a great heart.

One evening I noticed that I had a bump on my head, this was only one bump, that's all it was one bump. The next day I was scheduled to preach and I wanted to look my best so I decided to employ my mother's herbal remedy. It was about 8:30 p.m. so I decided that I would make up the oatmeal paste and apply it to my bump and then once the bump had shrank I was going to remove the oatmeal paste and go to sleep. I made up the oatmeal paste but it was kind of difficult to make up such a small amount so I decided just to make up enough oatmeal paste to put the paste all over my head. Maybe it would help to keep any future bumps away.

I made up the oatmeal paste and applied it all over my head. It was now about 9:00 p.m. and I was getting sleepy but I knew I couldn't lie down on the bed with all that oatmeal paste on my head, my wife would kill me. I decided to put a towel under my head but the oatmeal paste would have messed up the towel. I decided to put a plastic cap on my head to keep the oatmeal paste from messing anything up and it worked out fine. It was now about 9:15 p.m. and I decided that I would lie down for a while and get up at about 11 p.m. or so and wash the oatmeal paste off my head. I was so tired I just fell fast asleep with the oatmeal paste and the plastic cap on my head.

The next day I woke up and I smelled oatmeal cooking. I guessed my wife was making us breakfast but I looked over and saw that she was still in the bed fast asleep. I reached up and touched my head and felt the plastic cap and remembered what had happened. I rushed into the bathroom took off the plastic cap and saw that the oatmeal paste had cooked on my head! I quickly washed off the oatmeal paste and saw that my head was now a bright pink!! A bright pink, I had just cooked my head!! I had a pink, bright pink scalp with my black face. Now don't you know that was a sight to see!! Do you see how one small thing can cause such a big problem? How one little bump and one little decision to do something in a certain way can cause a big problem.

But I know what you are thinking and I bet the suspense is killing you. What you want to know is what happened to the bump? The small little bump that started all of this. Well the only good thing about all of this is that the bump was gone.

My mother had many different remedies that she had told me about during the course of her life. She is gone now and I do miss her so badly but I know where she is and I know that one day I will see her again and that eases the pain some but it was always fun talking to mom. But now back to the SUV.

As I waited in my big SUV for the police to arrive the pain in my back had intensified and I began to realize that this was a little more serious than I had thought. When the policemen arrived he asked both me and the driver of the other vehicle to sit in the back seat of the police car, while he took his report. My back was now feeling as if I had been; well as if I'd been in a car wreck. To make matters worse the seats that we had to sit on were made of hard molded plastic and were causing me considerable discomfort. As the policeman was finishing up his questions I was so relieved because the seats were so very uncomfortable.

As I walked back to my big SUV I looked at the tow truck moving the other driver's little car off the street. It had been rendered undrivable and would probably be totaled out. The front end of the other vehicle was almost totally destroyed. I do not see how the engine did not injure the occupants in that car.

But I think it may have had a transverse or side ways mounted engine.

I also learned that the other driver was driving in the curb lane while I was in the center lane. There was a car that was in front of him that stopped in front of him without signaling to make a right turn. To avoid hitting that car he pulled over into the center lane where my vehicle was. As he sped up to look over at the other driver he began blowing his horn and flipping the bird at the driver of that car. At that precise moment the car in front of me stopped, so I stopped. When he turned his head around he saw my stopped vehicle but was unable to avoid it. He estimated that he was doing about 45 to 50 mph when he made contact with my big SUV. That explained why the front of his vehicle received so much damage; he basically accelerated into the rear of my big SUV at 50 mph.

Proverbs 19: 21 reads " There are many devices in a man's heart; nevertheless the counsel of the Lord, that shall stand."

We may decide to plan many things in a certain way to achieve a desired result but no matter how precise and detailed our plans are God is the one who will get what he wants. As a leader of different organizations I have been required to be proactive in anticipation of many problems that could occur. It was necessary for me to develop emergency plans to address the possibility of fires, severe weather evacuation plans and many other plans.

When we decided to buy this big SUV my wife and I liked the way it's sat up high and seemed to be constructed very strong and powerfully. And if one-purchased accessories like Auto ride it helped to minimize the risks of rollover and provided a stable quiet ride. I think that had I been driving one of my other vehicles the damage to it would have been much greater. I also believe that I would have sustained much greater injuries as well. Our decision to buy this bigger more powerful vehicle; and I use the term OUR loosely, because generally wife's buy cars, husbands pay for them, had proven to be a good one because it had caused me to receive very little overall damage to my body. As a matter of fact the damage that I received seem to be a specifically located in my lower back and upper buttock areas.

The pain and the sensation that I was experiencing reminded me of a paddling that I had received when I was in school and had been disrespectful to my football team and had not represented them properly. I was going to play in my first varsity football game as a sophomore, as a varsity player I was required to wear the varsity blazer and a tie on game day. Just to make sure I'm not misunderstood we also had to wear shoes, a dress shirt and pants also. I didn't want you to think that we were nudist or heathens or anything. I was wearing the blazer but I didn't have on my tie, it was in my pocket.

One of my teachers and also one of my varsity football coaches, Coach Herbert Alvin asked me why I wasn't wearing a tie? Every time I say his name I get a little pain in my posterior gluteus maximus (ouch!!). I explained to Coach Herbert Alvin that my tie was in my pocket because it felt a little uncomfortable and I took it off for just a little while. That sounded like a good excuse to me, doesn't that sound like a good excuse to all you readers? The tie was a little bit tight and uncomfortable so I took it off. OK!! Sounded pretty good to me, doesn't that sound pretty good to you readers? But It Didn't Sound Good to Coach Alvin!!! As a matter fact it made him very angry. He got right up in my face, or as the kids would say today, all up in my grill, and said to me what do you mean a little uncomfortable; don't you know you're representing yourself, your classmates, your school, your team, and your coaches. What are you doing, trying to make us all look bad? Then he showed me how to put on the tie without it feeling uncomfortable at all. Leave your top button open and knot the tie tight but not to tight.

From now on I want you to wear your tie but to make sure you remember I want you to come out into the hall with me and I'm going to give you a little reminder. Coach Herbert Alvin gave me one SWAT; that SWAT was so hard that I call it the SWAT that was heard around the world but from that day on I remembered to wear my tie on game day. Sometimes painful experiences can be useful reminders to help us not forget important events. When we think about Jesus and how painful the price was that he paid for us and our salvation it's a reminder that we owe him so much and that we need to represent him to the best of our abilities. We have been bought with a price and that price was his blood that he shed for us on Calvary. What a fantastic God we serve. What a great savior he is. Back to my big SUV.

I was able to drive my big SUV away from the accident scene and as I did I couldn't help but think, what is God trying to tell me that he had to give me a spanking by hitting me in the back side with 2000 pound paddle? I knew that God was fair and that he would not deal with me in such a powerful manner unless there was a very important reason for him doing so. I was now asking myself what was I missing what did I need to do that God had taken this drastic action to get my attention. God does not allow correction to come or a disaster to strike without there being a very significant reason for its occurrence.

Sometimes we are in the forest so deeply that we cannot see the trees. But I knew that God had something that he wanted me to correct and change and I was ready to hear whatever he wanted to say and do whatever he wanted me to do. I was all ears and I just was ready to hear the Lord speak and I was hopeful that this situation could start changing and that I could get through whatever I needed to get through as quickly as possible. So that I could get back into living the kind of life that I wanted to live.

Now my positive thinking started to kick in. I told myself considering the amount of force that my big SUV had been hit with just to have the pain localized in my back area was a very good thing. As a matter of fact one could almost say that it was a blessing to only have that amount of damage done to me. I knew my body very well and I knew that it had responded and come back from many different injuries; ruptured Achilles' tendon, chipped bone on my femur, previous back injuries and other various injuries. I was very optimistic that I would have an extremely speedy recovery and that the pain in my butt and my back would be going away very soon. I estimated that in a week or at the most two this would all be a distant memory to me. I turned on my CD player and continued to listen to my gangster rap confident that I would be okay very soon. A little ice and a little heat and I'll be fine.

    I continued on to the funeral I got there and began to give my apologies for being late explaining that I was just in a car wreck and that I knew that I would be all right because God is greater than any little car. After the funeral was over and I was leaving the funeral home I noticed that my back felt Worse!!

Chapter 9

Hurry Up and Wait: On God

" Be still, and know that I am God: I will be exalted among the heathen, I will be exalted in the earth." (Psalms 46: 10)

One of the hardest things for us to do is wait on the Lord. When we come before God we want him to hurry up and do the things that we want done. We ask God for patience but we want to get that patience right now. We will even allow him to work on us, to change us and to mold us but we want him to operate on us and to do it right now. As Americans we want everything instantly and in a hurry. If we go out to dinner and our dinner is five minutes late then we want to see the manager and we're demanding that we get a discount or a free meal. If we start a new job on the lowest level, within a month we want to get a promotion, within six months we want to be managing the department and within a year we want to be one of the directors of the company. Within two years we want to become owners of our own businesses.

And do not let us start on a workout program even if we have to lose 500 pounds we think we ought to be able to lose that in two maybe three weeks at tops. If we do not look like Beyonce, Katherine Heigl, Mary-Louise Parker or Vanessa Williams if you're a woman or LL Cool J, Eric Dane, Jamie Foxx or Brad Pitt, if you're a man within a month then we think that the exercise program was a flop! Then we say something like I can't believe I put in all that time I work so long and hard to get such poor results. I'm just going to give up and go out to the buffet and eat my troubles away at least then I'll feel better.

Or we are so busy and in a hurry trying to get the better things in life that both parents are working two jobs. The kids are going to school and then are involved in extracurricular activities. They're playing soccer, or football in the fall, basketball in the winner, track in the spring and baseball in the summer. Mom and dad take turns running the kids to the different practices and games in between job commitments. Then the kids have school assignments and homework they must do so they must complete that. We add to that the time that we spend on the computer or on the cell phone or text messaging and there's no wonder that we say we don't have time to do anything.

We are just so impatient and in such a hurry that we don't really have time to appreciate all of the most important things in life. We are so busy that one parent is leaving home taking a group of kids somewhere while the other parent is returning home with a group of kids. We just pass each other like ships in the night. It's a wonder most parents have found enough time to make a family!! We're just so busy busy busy and so impatient impatient impatient. The only time we actually rest is when we have to, like when we get sick or when we become hurt and have to slow down.

Be still and know that I am God I'll be exalted among the heathen I'll be exalted in the earth. (Psalms 40:16) Stop all the running around, stop being impatient just be still be quiet, as the old people used to say, "be still and hush." God is telling us that he is Elohim, the mighty and powerful God and that there is no one on earth that is more powerful than him. We can relax and stop all of the busyness and rushing around that we are doing and just appreciate who he is.

When is the last time that we took out our Bible's, turned off the television, turned off the radio, turn off the computer, the cell phone and just read our Bible for 10, 15, 30 or more minutes. We don't let anything else interrupt us as we were reading about the goodness, the mercy, the grace and the power of God. As we do this it becomes a habit that we will find ourselves repeating many times over. Because there is nothing better on this earth than for a spirit filled Christian to have the opportunity to read about and experience the wonders of God as they are revealed in his word. And then we are also able to receive from God through his word the directions and instructions which we need to live the kind of life that he wants us to live.

Or how long has it been since we got on our knees, prayed to God and told him about our love for him and about how appreciative we are for being his children. Or talking to God in prayer about our troubles and about our problems. Letting him know what our fears and our cares are and knowing that he hears us and that he will always give us an answer. It may not be the answer that we want but he will always give us the answer that we need. The answer may not come in the time that we want it but it will be within the time that we need it.

When was the last time that we went off by ourselves to a quiet corner or place and just enjoyed being in the presence of God? Just relaxing and allowing the presence of God to flow over us like a gentle wave. Being totally and completely immersed in the presence of God, wholly and deeply absorbed in him. Having that special time of fellowship and worship with the Lord God knowing that he cares so much for us. Knowing that he loves to have fellowship with us as much as we enjoyed having fellowship with him.

Let's do ourselves a favor, at our earliest opportunity let's read the Genesis account of how God created and cared for man in the beginning. We will start at Genesis 1: 26 and we will conclude at Genesis 2: 25. We will see just how much God cared for and provided for man. We will see that man was and is the centerpiece of God's creation and that God had prepared an almost perfect environment for man. The only improvement that God made to this environment was to provide the addition of the woman who could only exist after the man was made because she had to come out of man. But I do not want us to read it right now but we need to read it later. That is the assignment that I am giving you so that you can see just how important we are to God and just how much God wants to fellowship with us because we are the Apple of God's eye. But now back to my big SUV.

I pulled my big SUV into my garage and went into the house. My wife whom I called earlier asked me how I was doing. I explained to her that I was hurting but that I would be fine because I knew what to do, (more positive thinking) I'd had physical problems before, I had conquered those and I will conquer this as well. I proceeded to begin ice therapy and rest for the rest of the day thinking that I would be ready to go the next morning. I also began positive affirmation, reciting to myself that my back would feel great tomorrow over and over again until I fell asleep. This was a technique that I used for years to program my mind to help me feel better in the morning and to help my overall feeling of well-being. I used it to perform well in athletic competitions and it worked so I started using this technique to help me in every aspect of my life.

The next morning I felt great pain in my middle and right lower back. It was extremely painful for me to get up out of the bed and make it to the bathroom. I also began to lean away from the pain and that gave me the appearance of a giant letter "C". I fought through the pain all the time thinking that it was not that serious and that the pain would go away very soon. I would "will" it out and work it out. I will be okay!! No little car like that was going to stop me. I leaned and limped my way to my garage to look at the little damage that was on the bumper of my big SUV to reassure me of the fact that that little damage should not be causing me all of this pain. I went back to my bathroom and showered determined to go about my day as usual. I was going to make my body ignore the pain and get better quickly; I had businesses to run and a ministry to launch, I didn't have time to be injured.

I got dressed as quickly as I could and went to my workout room to prepare for my workout. I have a very nice well-equipped workout room. It has a treadmill, an elliptical machine, heavy bag, speed bag, free weights, abs machine and an all in one lifting machine. As I attempted to stretch out my back I experienced even more pain but I kept on trying because I did not want to give in to the pain. The more I tried the greater the pain became, I realized that I was just irritating and aggravating the injury more. I looked around at all of my equipment and I told "it" that I would be back tomorrow, guaranteed.

The next day I got up and went through the same routine, the same pain, the same lean and limp scenario, only this time I had additional pain shooting down from the top of my right leg to my right foot. I tried to stretch and to work out with the same results. I decided to go to an emergency care facility to get examined and x-rayed. The doctor said he thought I had a severe back strain, he gave me a prescription for some pain killers (which I hate to take) but I was in so much pain I was glad to get it. He also told me to go see my orthopedic physician for follow-up. Well I guess this is going to take a little longer then I thought. But I'm glad that I know it is just a little back strain, I've had many strains, piece of cake, I'll be ready to go in a week or so. Let's go get those painkillers because my back is still killing me!!

I drove to the pharmacy in my big SUV and gave the pharmacist the prescription, when he came back with the pills I almost broke his wrist because I snatched them from him so fast. Apologizing I took a warm bottle of water off the shelf and began to guzzle down two of the pills, thank God that was the right dosage. I hate taking medication of any kind, I very seldom gets sick or have pain that I can't handle but isn't it funny how we act when we are dealing with unusual situations. When we are hurting in unusual ways we will seek unusual remedies. We'll look to anything and go any place to get help.

If we have experienced a loss or have some trouble in our lives that is causing us pain of any kind, we often tend to look for some way to anesthetize the hurt and the pain. In that instance some folks turn to drugs to ease the pain and the suffering that they are experiencing. Some folks will turn to illicit sexual liaisons to ease the pain of loneliness. And some will turn to overeating to try to fill a void or to resolve a problem. There is an old saying "it's not so much what you're eating, that makes you gain weight, it's what's eating you".

This could be the reason why we have so many obese people in our nation. They could be hurting or there could be a void in their lives and they are trying to fill it with food. If they would just turn their pain over to Jesus. If they would just turn the emptiness over to Jesus he would be able to stop their hurting and fill that void. He can make it all right. If you are hurting or you feel empty inside, call on Jesus he will satisfy all your needs.

I made the appointment with my doctor, he examined me and in his opinion, I had severe back strain that he thought would clear up in a little while. He prescribed some painkillers and muscle relaxants. This doctor had been my orthopedic physician for over 30 years and his opinion meant a lot to me. When he told me this I felt as if a great weight had been lifted off of me. I left his office feeling great mentally but I still had that pain in my back and leg. I limped and leaned over to my big SUV and speedily drove to the pharmacy to get those painkillers and muscle relaxants. Strange how quickly we can get used to something that we used to despise when it seems to ease our pain.

It had now been over 2 months since that little car hit my big SUV, I had not been able to run or lift as I used to, nor was I able to even walk very far and when I did it was extremely painful. Two different doctors, one who I had known me for over 30 years and that I trusted very much, had told me that it was just a small problem, a strain that should resolve itself very quickly. All of that was fine and dandy, but instead of feeling better, my back and leg were feeling worse!! I also notice something else I was starting to get out of breath when I was walking for short periods of time and was getting soft around my middle. I was starting to get a gut; I was getting out of shape. I leaned and limped to my bathroom, took off my clothes and weighed myself; in just 2 months I had gained 4 pounds.

Unable to run the 3-5 miles for five days a week and not lifting the 2 days per week that I normally did was starting to take its toll. Also because I was not as active as I normally was I was not moving around burning up the normal amount of calories than I should have. Another unwanted byproduct of the injury was the gnawing anxiety and fear of not seeing any results of getting better. This seemed to cause me to lean and limp to the refrigerator or the pantry nervously grabbing something to eat. Because of not being able to be as active as I had been I now had more time on my hands and I was filling it and my hands with food. Potato chips and miniature candy bars became my best friends. Something was wrong, this had to change this is not a typical strain there has to be something else going on.

I went back for the follow-up with my orthopedic physician and told him about the pain I was still experiencing. We decide to schedule an MRI of my back. The MRI revealed that I had two herniated discs and a synovial cyst on my spine. It felt good knowing what was wrong because now we could attack the problem and resolve it. The normal course of treatment was to take three injections to help shrink the cyst and block the pain from the discs. This should permit me to be able to function in a less painful state. Having been involved in athletics for many years I heard the horror stories about many players who had those injections and got relief for a short period of time only to have to get more injections later. It disguised the pain but didn't resolve the problem. This course of treatment finally resulting in long-term damage to the joint.

That was not for me, I wanted a long-term solution not just a temporary pain fix. We decided on a course of treatment that involved ice and heat therapy, stretching, anti-inflammatory medication and exercise. I explained to my doctor that my back felt as if I needed to be straightened out, as if I needed to be pulled to straighten it out. My doctor didn't know it but I had 2 friends of mine that weighed over 300 pounds and who were very strong and I was contemplating having one pull on my legs and the other on my arms to stretch me and straighten me out. Man was I desperate I just wanted the pain to stop and get back to my normal active life.

What desperate measures we will take to get restored back to a certain type of lifestyle that we thought was better for us?

If we were in the process of losing something, maybe a house which was going to be foreclosed on. Maybe a car that was going to be repossessed. Or a job that we had for a long time and now we were facing a layoff or the plant was shutting down. What would we do?

Or what about that long-term relationship that we have been in for over five years and now out of the blue, out of left field somewhere, without any warning, the other person wants to get out of the relationship. We thought that everything was fine and that there was nothing to be concerned about but now out of nowhere this comes up! Our head is spinning, thoughts are running at hyper speed through our mind. What am I going to do now, "who can we turn to when nobody needs us", where'd that come from, this is no time for songs I got to get myself together before I lose my mind. Lord just please hurry up and stop the pain, before I go crazy, what would you do to stop the pain?

I began asking God in prayer to please hurry up and reveal to me what I needed to correct and please do it quickly. I started thinking about these words, from Psalms 46: 10, "be still and know that I am God."

Chapter 10

Who Are You Going to Straighten Out? Who Do You Think Is In Charge Anyway?

"Consider the work of God: for who can make that straight, which he has made crooked? In the day of prosperity be joyful, but in the day of adversity consider: God also hath set the one over against the other, to the end that man should find nothing after him." (Ecclesiastes 7: 13 & 14)

All right it's time to get this show on the road and take control and get my physical and my mental life back! It's been almost 6 months now and it's time, I'm ready to go there ain't nothing that is going to stop me now, excuse my French but I'm ready to go, I'm excited! I went to see a chiropractor for about 15 visits but I got mixed results so I stopped that. The manipulation and heat felt pretty good but it didn't last and I went back to leaning and limping. I did like the tens machine and I think I'll buy one of those. I've been doing the exercises, which consists of stretching, light lifting and walking. I still have the pain in my lower back and leg but I do not want to take the shots that my doctor says should help.

I do have some periods of time when my leg does not hurt so that's encouraging with a little more dedication, perseverance and prayer this thing is going to start to turn around pretty soon. I have gotten back to reading my Bible more and that is a plus. Oh yeah, how could I forget I've gained about 15 pounds since this accident happened and I really don't like that at all. I used to feel that people who were overweight were just lazy and ate too much, which for some people that is true but not for everyone. Sometimes there are extenuating circumstances and situations which are beyond our control, but I bet if I would stop eating those potato chips and those miniature candy bars I probably would not have gained as much weight as I did.

It's been almost 18 months since my big SUV was rear-ended by that little car and I'm still having pain in my lower back and intermittently down my leg. It is not as bad as it was but I still lean and limp. I'm still continuing on with the heat, ice and exercise therapy. I've also bought a tens machine and have incorporated that into the treatment program. Because of a recent meditation scare I had to discontinue one of the medications (I am now on three) and was trying to function on those. I also am so glad that it's fashionable to wear these big hooded sweatshirts because they hide the extra 26 pounds I have now gained, and when I lean and limp it looks like I'm trying to be cool and pimp when I walk. I still haven't given in and taken the shots yet.

I really do not like the way I look with this extra weight and I've noticed that I have some physical side effects and some mental side effects from this extra weight. I've noticed that physically I find myself getting short of breath and I do not have the strength or the stamina that I've had most of my life. I am sleeping more than I ever have before, around 9 to 10 hours whereas before I slept 5 or 6 hours per day. I also noticed my vision seemed to be blurry and not as clear as before I gained this weight.

Mentally I never had a negative self-image and was always proud of my physique but I am now ashamed of the gut that I am carrying. I also have a spare tire around my waist and I don't like that either. I also am experiencing depression that I have never experienced before and a lack of self-worth and a feeling of helplessness. Being unhealthy or sick can really take a lot of confidence out of you. This has really been a very humbling experience for me. I never would've thought that I would be brought down to this level physically by that little car rear-ending my big SUV.

It's been 30 months since that little car rear-ended my big SUV and I really cannot believe it's been that long. Here I am lying on my stomach in the hospital preparing to receive the second shot in my back to relieve the pain. My doctor told me that sometimes the first shot doesn't work and you need to take a second and sometimes a third shot for them to be effective. Well here I am the guy said he wouldn't take any of those shots with his gluteus maximus in the air getting ready to be stuck again. It's amazing what we will do when we become desperate and are hurting isn't it, amen.

I have gained 30 pounds, my breathing has become labored my knees are hurting from carrying the extra weight, my eyes are still blurry, mentally I still feel the depression and the helplessness and my back & leg have improved but they still are hurting. The last shot lasted for about seven days but it did feel good hopefully this one will last as promised, about six months or more.

I hope that this works to make my crooked back straight. I have tried and done many things that I said I would not do. I have always been very hesitant to take any drugs or medications but during the last 30 months I have taken several different drugs, one of which has been responsible for the death of several of the individuals who took it. I have also sought medical help from many different practitioners and have used their advice in an attempt to resolve this problem. But as of yet I have not found any solution that has been able to resolve this problem and to give me any lasting relief.

It's almost as if there is something that is preventing all of the best efforts and plans which I have employed and the doctors and therapists have tried to be effective. I know that God is sovereign and is in control of everything but for the life of me I really do not understand what I may have done to have caused this, or why I need to have this type of correction or lesson. In the past I have never asked God why me because I knew that he is just and fair and has always provided me with a better outcome than I deserved.

But I wish that I could hear from God soon so that he can let me know what I need to do to turn this situation around. Why has such a little thing turned into something so big and caused me so much pain and suffering for so long? If I could just have a little talk with him and find out what he wants me to do. I would do it in a heartbeat so that this pain and suffering could come to an end. If he could just provide me with a solution, a remedy for this problem I would implement it without hesitation. I know I said I should be still and know that God is God but man when one is suffering and in pain it's hard very hard to be still. Well it's time for my shot; I hope it works better than the last one.

It is now 36 months since that little car rear-ended my big SUV and it's been 6 months since I tried that injection to help reduce my back pain. The shot lasted for about eight days and then the pain returned as strong as ever. My doctor had put me on exercise limitations that called for no running, no heavy lifting, no fast bending, no sudden twisting and turning. The hope was that this shot would alleviate the pain and allow me to resume some of my former activities. I had tried to run and that really cause my back to give me excruciating pain. After telling my doctor about the pain we had decided to seek help from one of the leading healthcare organizations in the world.

I was then referred to one of the leading teams that specializes in back care and rehabilitation in the world. This team consisted of approximately 10 different doctors who had various approaches they would employ to help me resolve my back problem.

The first doctor on the team examined me and reviewed my MRI and suggested that I try to forget about my back problems and just began to try to do some of the former things I had done including running. He said that he had pain medications that he could prescribe that would help me exist almost in a pain-free state. He was talking to me, the guy who had hated taking medication 3 years earlier about these super powerful medications. I bet you know what I told him don't you? I told him sure let's try those super powerful medications; I was still so desperate by now I would try anything. To make a long story short these painkillers didn't help my back. When I tried to exercise, especially when running, the pain was excruciating. We tried on 2 other occasions to increase my activities but did not have any better results. When I told the doctor this he referred me to another doctor on the team.

This doctor examined me and reviewed my MRI and told me that there was a procedure that could be performed on my back in which the nerves could be removed or burned away in that area with a very fine instrument and I would not be able to feel the sensation of pain in that area. To my way of thinking the reason why God had allowed us to have nerves in that area was because he wanted us to feel things in that area and if the nerves were burnt away we probably wouldn't be able to do that. I also did not want to take the chance of them burning up some other things that I might need back there. I really didn't want to be roasted or toasted back there. This doctor referred me to the best doctor on the team.

This doctor examined me and reviewed my MRI and told me that he had a procedure that he used that would help remove most or all of the pain that was going down my leg. However he could not guarantee that the pain in my back would cease after this procedure. He said that the pain in my back could be coming from many different sources and he could not guarantee that they would be able to find the source but that he could with reasonable certainty eliminate most of the pain which was running down my leg. He said he had this kind of Ream-Rooter process that he used to open up the area so that the nerves would have more room to function. I told him that I had to have some time to think about it and I would get back with him.

Yeah, right, sure I was going to let him do a Ream-Rooter process on me. I decided right then and there that it was time for me to do what I should have done so long ago. As soon as this accident had happened I should have went straight to God in my private closet and began to seek his face. I should have asked him what he wanted me to do and what I needed to correct in my life that had caused him to permit such a small thing to balloon and grow into such a large problem. I should have went to God and threw myself on his mercy and his grace and just asked him to forgive me for whatever I had done and to cleanse me from all the unrighteousness that was in my life. The Bible tells us in *Isaiah 64: 6 "But we are all as an unclean thing, and all our righteousness are as filthy rags; and we do all fade as a leaf; and our inequities, like the wind have taken us away."*

It does not matter how clean and righteous we think we all are or how clean and righteously we think we are all living we are all as filthy rags in the presence of our holy God. Because we all have unclean and unholy minds even when we think we are doing the right thing and thinking the right way. Why? Because we are processing our thoughts through our unholy and unclean minds we can still deceive ourselves. We can justify our own actions because we will hold everyone else to a higher standard. When we are dealing with ourselves we will lower those same standards to accommodate and facilitates our own sinful ways.

We need to get down on our knees and forget about all of the façades, which we have put up, the many different masks that we put on and the many different faces that we put on. The many different disguises that we use to cover up who we really are and just go before God and get flat on our faces and asked him to search us, to cleanse us, to hold us, to comfort us, to instruct us, to chasten us, to correct us, to guide us and finally to restore us.

Chapter 11

Do You Really Want to Hear? Do You Really Want to See?

" I have heard of thee by the hearing of the ear: but now my eye seeth thee. Wherefore I abhor myself, and repent in the dust and ashes."(Job 42:5-6)

I got down on my knees and I began to seek God's face and I just wanted to enter into his presence and feel the fellowship of his Holy Spirit. To feel the security and safety of his closeness and his embrace. To finally feel his loving arms around me and knowing that I was not there to get anything but what he wanted to give me. Have you ever come to God with an agenda, with the hope of telling him what you wanted from him but now you're just so happy to be in his presence that you forget all about your list and are ready to hear what he has to say to you. You're ready to take his list, his requests. And then he opened up the veil and showed me what I really looked like, what I could look like and what I needed to do to become who he had called me to become.

 The feeling of being secure and comforted had been replaced with a feeling of fear and anxiety. The kind of feeling you use to get when you were about to be disciplined or scolded for doing something that you knew you should not have done. And you knew that you had no defense or any hope of changing the mind

Coming Alive At 55

of the one who was going to provide the discipline because you knew that you deserved every bit of punishment that you were about to get.

In the spirit I could hear God say: You walked away from the Ministry almost 10 years ago and you said you were coming back but you never did. I called you to the Ministry and when you answer you were so happy and so was I. I knew what was inside of you and how you could battle and fight for me. But you got discouraged and decide to walk away without so much as checking with me. I gave you a great helpmate someone who completes you and who has helped you in many great ways. You didn't even talk with her about it to get her viewpoint; she may have been able to help you after all that's what good helpmates do. I provided you with access to many different platforms and equipped you to fit in anywhere you would go. And you took it as if it was just your abilities and your training that provided access to all the things that I provided for you. I have protected you from so many dangers that you would not even have enough fingers and toes to count them and you feel that you were the one who did it.

I have blessed you and have graced you with so much prosperity and health that you just took it for granted as if you had the Midas touch. You thought that there was nothing that you could not accomplish and that anything you put your hand to would work out the way you wanted. But I am the one who blessed you with favor and provided you with a life of ease. Do you really think that you could have done all those things on your own? You told so many people that it was God and that if they trusted in him they too could achieve if they just have faith, but I gave you so much you did not have too have any faith because everything you wanted was already there. I would even give you something as small and mundane as a parking space in the spot you wanted and I did it so often that you took that for granted. And now you don't even want to say a few words for me. How ungrateful and selfish you are.

I have proved so many times that I love you because loving is giving and I've given you so much. Sure you give people money but how many of them have you given yourself to? When is the last time that you told someone about me or my son or my Holy Spirit? You used to be so on fire for me that you would get up every morning and study my word, not just read as you had been doing lately but you would study my word. When you were running on the tread-mill you would read my words as you ran just to sincerely show how you loved me and because you wanted to spend more time with me. You would have your radio turned on to the Christian stations and you would wake up to someone preaching my word every day. Then you would go out and tell someone about me and my son and my holy spirit and how special you knew that we were.

I felt so good and so important when you would tell people about us. I love to come around those who praise me because this world is praising me less and less these days. But it won't be long before my son will be coming back and every knee shall bow and every tongue shall confess that he is Lord!! But what I want to know is when are you going to start acting like someone who has already bowed down on his knees and confessed with his mouth that I am Lord of his life and when are you going to start really telling somebody about us.

When is the last time that you fasted just for me, to become closer to me and to clean up your life? When are you going to show me the same sacrificial love that I have shown you? The music that you have been listening to lately, this gangster rap, get rid of it now, garbage in garbage out! Some of those movies that you've been going to see, they are just a waste of our time; we have so little time, and so much work to do, stop wasting our time. I want you to clean up your mouth and your conversation, how can you a man of God, dare use your mouth to say words like those! I was now crying uncontrollably feeling ashamed and embarrassed for the way I had been behaving. *"But I say unto you, that every idle word that men shall speak, they shall give account thereof in the day of judgment, for by thy words thou shall be justified and by thy words thou shall be condemned."*(Matthew 12: 35-36). How many of us are going to places that we should not go, not bad places just not the best places and we're just hanging out wasting our time? Or how many of us are saying things that are not bringing any glory to God and are really showing him great dishonor and disrespect? Everything we say or do God hears and sees.

Look at your body!! Look at how fat and out of shape you are!! Sure you've been hurt but you didn't need to eat all of those bad foods. Eating all those potato chips and candy bars, please, filling the void you have for me with them, pleeeaaaseee. You've been working out all your life you know what to do. And I expect you start telling others about what you know. Do you really want to hear what I have to say? Do you really want to see what you look like to me and what you could look like to me?

I'm am the one true God, full of love, grace and mercy but I am also a jealous God full of wrath, justice and righteousness; and I want to know if you really want to hear me and see me? I felt so unworthy and filthy but I knew that he was right and that I needed to hear what he was saying to me. I need to tell you that you have been acting self-righteous and arrogant, as if you are above those people that I called you to help and to serve. Now that you have been going through your physical and mental changes it's kind of knocked you down a peg or two hasn't it? It knocked you off your high horse didn't it? When you didn't have the go through anything it was easy to look down and judge others but now because you went through something instead of judging you have sympathy for them. Instead of judging now you want to pray for them and show them how to do things don't you. You've been humbled now haven't you? At anytime I choose I can bring you to your knees. And no one can get you off of them but me!!! I am Yahweh, The All Mighty One of oaths.

Let me explain something to you, the reason why I sent my son to come to earth in human form was so that he, who was so far above you, could come and tell you and show you how I wanted you to live. My son had every right to look down upon you but instead he served you, showed you how to live, loved you and then he died for you. But that is how I do things, I take those who know what to do and I have them teach those who do not know what to do. Someone had to teach you didn't they? Do you think that you were just born into the knowledge that you have? Did you just get it out of thin air? I started to answer but God said Shut up I'm Not through Speaking yet!!

You must <u>Remember What Your Mother Asked You to Do And Do It! And you also must remember to do what you knew you were supposed to do in your heart!!! You have been talking about and thinking about retirement, Retirement!! You are only 54 years old!! Moses was almost 80 when he led my people from the bondage of Egypt. Retirement, you and so many of your generation are stop working just when you're starting to figure things out. You're stopping just when you're starting to get some sense about what's going on in life. Retirement, I've given you 54 years to do what you wanted to do, Now Its Time for You to Do What I called you to do & what I want You to Do. It's time for you to come alive!</u>

<u>It's time for you to wake up from your 54-year slumber!! It's time for you to come alive at 55, come alive at 55, come alive at 55</u>

If you do I will give you rest from the pain but like Paul, you will occasionally have a thorn in the flesh as a reminder of your past failures, your selfish attitude and my power and might; but I want you to know that my grace is sufficient for thee for my strength is made perfect in weakness. The weaker you become the stronger I will become in you and you will be able to preach my word and do my will. When you do I will let you again know the true joy of my fellowship and salvation. You will then experience the peace that comes from doing my work and abiding in my will. If you do it right than I will give you long life also! Only I know how long you will live!

I no longer felt the presence of fear and anxiety but now I felt a calmness and a peace that was far better and exceeded by far any feeling of peace that I ever felt before. It truly was a peace which goes beyond all understand and no matter how hard I tried I couldn't find any words to describe the feeling that washed over me. I was now crying uncontrollably but I didn't feel unworthy anymore I didn't feel filthy anymore. With every tear I could feel the cleansing power of the Holy Spirit washing over me cleansing me from the filth of arrogance. Cleansing me from the filth of self centered living and self righteousness; removing the spirit of judgment and condemnation, liberating me to be able to start fresh and clean with a brand-new attitude of servant hood and love. Wanting to help all the people I encounter in whatever way I can and in whatever way God wants me to.

I've been thinking about retirement just taking it easy and doing the things that I wanted to do in life, but I realized that it was no longer an option because now I have a new clear understanding about the power of God, the sovereignty of God, the will of God and the fact that what God wants he will get. We may have our own plans and our own agendas that we might think that we can submit to God and he would just sign off on whatever it is that we decide to do but that is not how it works at all. We are told in the book of Jeremiah 18:4-6

> *" And the vessel that he made of clay was marred in the hand of the potter: so he made it again another vessel that seemed good to the potter to make it then the word of the Lord came to me saying, O house of Israel, cannot I do with you as this potter? Saith the Lord. Behold, as the clay is in the potter's hand, so are ye in my hand, O house of Israel."*

In these verses we see the illustration that just as a potter can take a piece of clay and begin to shape and mold it into a certain form. If he is not happy with the original form because it did not come out the way that he had wanted it to. The potter can take the clay he was unhappy with and he can reform and reshape it and make it into a form that he is happy with. That is exactly what God wants to do with us if we have not been performing the way that he wants us to perform. He is going to reshape our lives to conform to the shape that he wants. But just as the clay did not put up a fight or resist the reshaping and reforming of the potter, we must be submissive and not resist God as he begins to reform us into the type of people that he wants us to become.

God wants to reform and transform us to equip and empower us to go up to the highest levels of our existence and to be able to achieve our full potential.

> *"And be not conformed to this world but be ye transformed by the renewing of your mind that ye may prove what is that good, and acceptable, and perfect will of God."(Romans 12: 2))*

This world tells us that as we become older the world wants to throw us away and just have us go over to the side and slowly fade out of the picture. And we tend to help them in their quest to have us fade away by retiring and just heading off into the sunset. I know of many individuals who have retired from successful careers just because they got tired of the job temporarily and wanted to do something else. Only to find themselves working menial jobs that they did not like and that were worse than the ones they left. So if you have a great job or career find something new and exciting to do on that job or find a great new hobby. Don't just quit because someone says you're old enough to retire but you still can have great income and security from the position or you still enjoy your work. Keep the money honey and learn how to fly a plane if you need more excitement but don't quit or retire unless you really want to!! Your not old your Vintaged!

God wants to take us out of that mindset, even if we are successful and have done what many folks call "made it" and we don't need to try to do anything else because we are successful on all levels that we operate on. We still can decide to do other things to challenge ourselves and to allow ourselves to grow into the kinds of individuals that God wants us to become. If we have been fortunate enough to be successful in life then we need to pass on our wisdom and our knowledge to help those who are less fortunate or less knowledgeable then we are. Decide to train someone or show someone how to become successful in life.

Become a mentor to someone or to a group of people. Find some way to give something back for all that God has given you and you truly will be able to come alive at any age especially at 55.

I started to feel better and lose some weight and the more weight I lost the better I felt. You know how good it feels when someone compliments you about the way you look and they say things to you like, you look great, whatever you have been doing? Keep it up. So I started complimenting myself and inspiring myself, spurring myself on to bigger and better results. The more I encouraged myself the better I did.

Sometimes you just have to encourage yourself, if you feel like you just can't make it and you're down and out, just start to encourage yourself and say positive things to yourself. Don't tear yourself down; you have enough negativity in your life already. Began to speak empowering and encouraging things to yourself to help build yourself up. You will be surprised at how quickly you will begin to feel better.

I felt better but I still leaned and limped, not quite as badly but it was still there and I still had pain. I know I had heard God correctly that he was going to give me rest from the pain and that I would only have occasional pain, but to date I had not received any rest from the pain. Then God brought a word to me that has changed my life and started me on the road to recovery, that word, that wonderful pain relieving life-changing word was traction.

I scheduled an appointment to see my doctor and when I went in to see him I asked him about traction. He said that if we would try it, it shouldn't hurt anything and what did we have to lose anyway? He said the new units were more powerful than the old ones and that if traction were going to work we would know very soon. My doctor scheduled the traction sessions and I could not wait until I would go to my first session. I went to my first session and almost immediately I could feel the pain ease and my crocked back began to straighten out. Within 3weeks I was feeling so much better and the pain in my back was gone!!

But the interesting thing about the traction is that I have to undergo a session every two weeks otherwise the pain will return. What an interesting reminder and thorn in the flesh. We tried a portable traction unit and found that it worked very well so I was able to now perform my traction therapy at home. But I am just so thankful for the periods of time when the pain is gone. The pain that used to run down my leg is almost nonexistent and I very rarely ever feel it. The pain in my back is also almost all gone when I do the traction once a week I have almost no incidents of pain. God could've made it so that I would have had to go to an external source to do my traction therapy but he provided me with a home unit so that I could do it at home.

I was now able to start thinking about running again and doing some light lifting without the excruciating pain that I had from the injury! Now I just had to go through the pain of getting back in shape but I was so happy that I would be able run and lift almost pain free! I started to walk and just to make it back on the treadmill was a great thing and I made it without any pain. Without any pain!!! I was walking pain free, next step, running!!

What a wonderful and great God we serve! He was willing to show me what I was lacking and he did it in the way that I really needed to be shown. God knows how to communicate with us in the language that we will understand and he knows how long to put us under that pressure so that we will do what he wants us to do. But he also knows when we've had enough and he will not put us under more pressure than we can bear. God is not a sadist who enjoys punishing us. He only does what is necessary to make us compliant or soften us up to do his will.

In the book of Jonah the story of his disobedience to God is recorded in chapters 1 and 2. God had wanted Jonah to go preach to the people of Nineveh, but Jonah decided he was not going to do it and ran away from God. Jonah got on a ship to get away but God caused a very violent storm to come up and violently rocked the ship. The sailors on the ship knew that God had caused the storm and they discovered that Jonah was the reason for it. The sailors threw Jonah overboard and God had prepared a big fish to swallow him.

The story tells us that Jonah was in the belly of the fish for three days and three nights until he finally agreed to go and preach to the people of Nineveh. When he agreed to do that the Bible says that the Lord spake unto the fish and it vomited out Jonah. Once Jonah had learned his lesson and had been softened up enough to do the will of God, God allowed the punishment to cease. That is exactly what he will cause to happen in our lives if we are disobedient to him. God will discipline us but once we've learned our lesson he will not continue to punish us. But we must truly repent & turn from our sinful ways.

It is now clear to me that he wants me to do something and I am ready to do it. I'm just so thankful and grateful to God that he has blessed me with my health. I also have a new desire, a new zeal, and a new fire to do what God wants me to do and I am happy to do it!! I feel like God has brought me back from the grave, back from the dead and he has allowed me to have a second chance at a new and vital life full of excitement and anticipation which comes from being available and ready to do what it is that he would have me to do.

I feel like shouting at the top of my lungs that I am so glad to be alive and that I am so grateful to God for giving me another chance for giving me a new life! Every day seems to be an exciting new adventure just waiting to happen just for me and God is the one who has made this all possible. But he can also do the same for you because he is no respecter of persons, what he has done for me he can do for you!

I will be more than happy to walk you through the process that I used to feel so good and I want to make this available to everyone who will read my story on how I was able to come alive at 55.

Are you ready? Are you ready? Are you ready to come alive at 55?

Chapter 12

Too Mature to Be Fat! Too Vintaged to Look Like That!

As my mother and I would go to the different funerals of our loved ones and our friends I would often tell her that there were four keys to living a long and healthy physical life. I told her that these keys would be worth more than gold to anyone who would first of all hear them and then began to apply them to their lives. And my mother would always tell me that somebody needs to tell everyone about these four keys as to allow them to have a great and healthy physical existence. After getting a physical the four keys are:

1. Get the right kind of rest, 6-8 hours of sleep per night.
2. Eat the right kinds of foods, fruits and vegetables and lean cuts of meat, chicken, fish, ect.
3. Exercise 30 to 40 minutes per day, walking is great but whatever exercise you do if it involves moving the big core muscles of your body it is good for you.
4. Don't put substances in your body that are bad for you, cigarettes, drugs, the wrong kinds of foods, alcohol etc.

I began to evaluate myself and to determine what I needed to do to reach the mental and physical fitness levels that I wanted to achieve. As I took a baseline of my mental condition I realize that I had been doing a lot of negative speaking and thinking toward myself. So I knew that the most important thing I had to do was to begin to speak positively into my life. So I began to tell myself good things about myself and how I was going to look better and better everyday. Just as the angel of the Lord had called cowardly Gideon a mighty man of valour, (Judges 6: 12) I was using positive affirmation to build myself up.

I began programming my mind again and I started thinking positive thoughts again. Just before falling asleep and getting my 6 hours of sleep, I would tell myself that I was going to be all right and that every day I was becoming stronger and better than I was the day before. I would recite over and over the phrase I'm going to feel great tomorrow, I'm getting better and stronger, my back feels great. We need to build ourselves up and fortify ourselves because we will become enthusiastic and confidence in the things that we are doing. When we become good at something we will also enjoy it more and look forward to doing it. Have you ever notice when we can do something well that sometimes we get so confident that we have to guard against becoming cocky and bragging on what we are able to do. So build yourself up but don't start bragging on yourself.

Slowly I could feel my attitude changing; those feelings of depression and negative self-image were slowly fading away. It was not an easy battle because the accuser of the saints, the devil, would always try to drag me back down into the pit of depression and self-loathing. But with continued prayer, positive thinking, listening to messages by men and women of God, such as T.D. Jakes, Joyce Meyers, Bill Winston, Paula White, Dr. Fred Price, R.A. Vernon, Pat Robertson, Joel Osteen and others was very helpful in renewing my positive attitude. I tried to immerse myself in their messages daily and they became great sources of encouragement and inspiration.

There is an old saying; if you show me your friends I will show you your future. I don't know who said it but it's so true, if you associate with people who are negative and are not positive influences on your life then you find yourself becoming negative and depressed. But if you have positive, upbeat and encouraging people in your life you will find those same qualities rubbing off on you and you will become like that also. So I decided even if it was through their messages and the media that these were some of the most positive, upbeat and encouraging friends that I could surround myself with. I did that and I am not sorry that I did. If you're going through something and need encouragement I recommend that you do the same thing. Find good positive influences to surround yourself with and it will improve your life and your attitude.

Reading Bible scriptures that promoted the power that God has and that we as his children also have, was very beneficial in reassuring me of the security which God provides for us and enabled me to be encouraged and strengthened daily. Scriptures such as *1st. John 4: 3 that reads "Ye are of God, little children, and have overcome them: because greater is he that is in you, than he that is in the world."*

When we read this Scriptures we are encouraged to believe that we can overcome anything because God has placed inside of us something that is greater than anything that we will face in this world. We are an overcomer and when we face any challenge no matter what it is we can overcome it!

I would read *Romans 13:1 "Let every soul be subject unto the higher powers, for there is no power but of God: the powers that be are ordained of God.* "This verse made it clear that God was in control of everything and that he is the source of all the powers that exists. God is in control of those powers and that if he decided that he is not going to provide power to something that it would be powerless. Therefore we do not have to fear anything that may come against us because God rules over that power and he can shut it off at any time. What A Mighty And Powerful God We Have As Our Protector And Provider!

I noticed that when I was anxious, depressed or upset the first thing that I would do is head for the refrigerator and medicate myself with food. Often times when I became emotional about something I would head for the potato chips and the miniature candy bars. So I started to get more control of my emotions by reading verses like this, *"For God has not given us the spirit of fear; but of power, and of love, and of a sound mind." 2nd. Timothy 1:7* Fear is defined in the dictionary as being afraid or frightened of something, to be uneasy or apprehensive about something, a feeling of anxiety caused by a real or and imagined danger. According to health.com about 3% of the U.S.A. population is faced with anxiety and fear attacks. We have panic attacks, acute stress disorders, general anxiety attacks, phobias, terror attacks, fear attacks and many more phobias that we suffer from and none of these are from God.

If God has not given us this spirit of fear then it must have been Satan that wants us to be fearful. Now I don't know about you but I don't want anything that Satan wants to give me. So I started to reject the spirit of fear that came from Satan and I began to accept and believe that I had the power and a sound mind that came from God.

I began to reclaim some discipline and self control again and the Lord gave me some very interesting thoughts. He asked me this question; has anyone ever showed up in your kitchen during your meal times with a gun and forced you to eat any of those foods that you have been eating? Has anyone ever put a spoonful of food into your mouth that you did not ask for or willingly accepted? I saw you when you were even trying to pray the calories out of a piece of chocolate cake and a bowl of ice cream!

You have even resorted to blaming the devil for making you get those potato chips and miniature candy bars. You're supposed to be a man of God with power and might saying that you are going to have the victory over the devil and you mean to tell me that you're not even strong enough to beat a potato chip and a miniature candy bar! Pleeeaaassee!!

I stopped my nervous eating and I began to eat only when I was hungry. I would eat breakfast, because it is a good way to start my metabolism for the day and to give me some energy. I would have cold cereal with skim milk or fruits and vegetables or oatmeal. Once in awhile I would have pancakes, and syrup or waffles or yogurt. For lunch I had salads, chicken, or fish sandwiches, fruit or vegetable bowls or a turkey sandwiches.

For dinner I have rice or a baked potato or a salad with fish or chicken, and once in a while I'd splurge and have a couple slices of pizza. I also would have an in between snack of a fruit smoothie whenever I wanted. I also ate fruits as an in between meal snack whenever I wanted to. Occasionally I also ate small portions of whole grain pasta.

I started drinking more water, about 8 to 10 8-ounce glasses of water daily. I got a product to help clean out my colon and to help me to remove the toxins from my system. Elimination is just as important as eating is or as my mother used to put it, honey the bathroom is just as important as the kitchen. There are many of us that are not so much overweight as we are just full of waste. We need to have regular stools to eliminate some of that waste that we have in us. There have been many stories and reports about people who have died and had autopsies performed upon them and it was discovered that they had 5 or 10 or 15 pounds of undigested waste in their colons. This waste is the source of many sicknesses and diseases and it is necessary to eliminate it from our system for good health. Death begins in a colon that is full of toxic waste.

I was really beginning to feel a lot better about the things that I had achieved so far and the progress that I had made encouraged me. But as of yet I had not faced the biggest challenge that I was going to have to encounter, the one that the doctors had said I would not be able to do, that was to run on the treadmill.

The last time I tried to run on the treadmill I had encountered excruciating pain. The reason that the doctors had said I should not do it was because the jarring and the pounding would cause my back to become misaligned, irritated and sore. But I knew that God had said he would give me rest from my pain and that I would only have it occasionally and I believed him. I knew if there was anyone that I could trust it was God the Father, God the Son, and God the Holy Spirit. I knew that I would be able to do it and I begin to prepare for my big test. To run on the treadmill!

In the book of Matthew Chapter 17 starting with verse 15 and concluding in verse 21 there is a story told about a man's son who was a lunatic or mental illness. The spirit that had possessed him would throw the son in the fire and in the water. I guess the spirit was trying to burn him up for a little while and then the spirit would put him out because the text said he did it often. He'd burn him for a while then put him out, burn him-put him out. So you can understand why his father was so distressed and was seeking help from Jesus' disciples. But his disciples were not able to cure him. Jesus answered in *verse 17 "O faithless and perverse generation, how long shall I be with you? How long shall I suffer you? Bring him hither to me. And Jesus rebuked the devil; and he departed out of him: and the child was cured from that very hour. Then came the disciples to Jesus apart, and said why could not we cast him out? And Jesus said unto them, because of your unbelief: for verily I say unto you, if ye have faith as a grain of mustard seed, ye shall say unto this mountain, Remove hence to yonder place and it shall remove; and nothing shall be impossible unto you. Howbeit this kind goeth not out but by prayer and fasting." (Matthew 17: 15-21)*

Jesus told his disciples that they needed to have faith, a strong prayer life and do some fasting and they would be able to achieve and accomplish anything! We could even cause a problem as big as a mountain to be removed from our lives if we have the faith, the prayer life and have been fasting. Do you have a big problem in your life something that has been plaguing you for quite awhile and you just don't know how to overcome it. Jesus has given us a great example and a tremendous blueprint that we can use to overcome any problem that we may encounter. How many of us know people who have struggled with drug addictions, sexual addictions, food addictions, and any of the addictions that could be treated successfully with this method.

If you're in a treatment program now don't stop but tell your doctor that you want to use this method alongside or hand-in-hand with your treatment program, but follow his advice. I'm sure if he is a good doctor he will not have any problem with you trying the faith, prayer and fasting method of Dr. Jesus.

I begin my preparation for my fast by eating salads, fruits, juices and water for three days slowly cutting out the salads and fruits. I began my fast of juices and water on the fourth day; I would enter into prayer and ask God to cleanse me of my sins, direct and guide me in my life and strengthened and fortify me to be able to accomplish his will. As I fasted I discover closeness to God and an intimacy that I had not experienced in quite some time. I also begin to feel the Holy Spirit in me become stronger and more vital as my flesh began to become weaker. I could just feel the Holy Spirit's energy flowing through me.

I started to evaluate where God had brought me from in just a little over 3 years. He has allowed me to grow so much and learn so much and has enhanced my knowledge and my understanding that I believe that we can achieve anything no matter what our age. Some folks think that when you become more mature and you pass the double nickel mark, you're supposed to have a big gut, a huge butt, big fat thighs and quadruple chins. I think that we know too much, that we are too experienced, that we have too much knowledge, that we know better, and that we are too mature to be fat!! We are too "vintaged" to treat ourselves like that.

The dictionary defines vintage as being of "extremely high quality!" How can we treat our precious, valuable, high quality self's in such a poor and disrespectful manner by allowing ourselves to become fat, overweight and out of shape. We are better then that and we can do better than that. We wouldn't let a gorilla drive our Lexus or Jaguar! We wouldn't dress a baboon in Armani, or put a set of Guirlande d'Ivioire linens in a doghouse so why are we mistreating our precious bodies?

What we must do is apply the things that we know and we will become capable of achieving weight control and good health without any problems. We must develop a plan and the discipline to adhere to that plan and this will allow us to accomplish our goal. Because we really are just too mature, we really do know too much and we really do know better than to be fooled by the things that we are being fooled by; those things that are causing us to gain the weight that we have and to exist in the poor physical state that we are in.

What profit is it to us to have education, position, power, properties and money if we don't have our health? If we don't have our health we don't have anything? Let's make up our minds to do all we can to improve our health and come alive with a new attitude of feeling and looking the best that we can! We may be older but that doesn't mean we can't get better! We are special, we are unique, we are not through and we are not dead. We are alive, We are alive, We are alive at **55**!!!!

Memo from Dr. M. D. Brown, 1st.
Who Knows How Long Any Of Us Will Live? If We Live to Be A 110 Years Old We Are Only Half Way There! What Will We Do With The Next 55 Years? Come Alive Now!!

Chapter 13

Keep Your Eyes Open And Your Knees Bent!

"Watch and pray, that ye enter not into temptation, the spirit indeed is willing, but the flesh is weak." (Matthew 26: 41)

Sometimes our bodies and our minds can play tricks on us. We may have a speech that we may have to give or an oral presentation that we are scheduled to do and we think that we will be fine. No problem just let me know when it's my turn to go and I'll be ready, I'm going to Ace this thing, I'm going to knock it out of the ballpark. Then the day of the presentation comes and we get up before all those people and cannot even remember our own names let alone what the presentation was to be about. Or we may have a date with someone and we are fine until we start walking down the sidewalk to their house, when we knock on the door and it opens our knees start knocking and we become tongue-tied. We aren't even able to say hello because we are so nervous.

What we must do is make sure that we are on guard against our flesh, to make sure it does not betray us and prevent us from doing what it is we are trying to do. That is why we must pray to God for the strength, energy and the power to control the flesh. Because the flesh is weak and tends to be easily influenced by outside stimuli, we must have a strong spirit that can control it. That is what's so great about fasting; it is the perfect way for us to further weaken the flesh and to fortify the spirit. As we go deeper into our fast we also develop a closer relationship with our heavenly father. We are less connected with and dependent upon the physical elements of our being and we are now relying more on God and his spirit to provide the guidance and power that we need to accomplish his will in our lives.

When we fast and deny ourselves of food which is something that we need to be able to live and survive, in an effort to come closer to God, that gets God's attention. God then starts to work with us to help and strengthen us and to give us the direction and leadership that we need to become better Christians. He gets on our side and is able to take us up to a new supernatural level of living that allows us to do more than we ever could before. During this time we are living less on our own physical power and more on the power of the Holy Spirit. Our spirit is now controlling our flesh with supernatural power.

I had been praying, reading my Bible and fasting and I was now ready to run on the treadmill. I also had been doing the traction and other physical therapy to help prepare my body to be able to run again. I knew that I was ready to face this mountain of a treadmill that was before me. I thought about all the times that I had come down in the past before I was injured and had effortlessly ran many miles on the treadmill before without any pain. Isn't it amazing how we can take something for granted until we are unable to have it or do it? A job that we had gotten tired of and decided to quit it but once it was gone we sure missed it. Or that husband or wife that we couldn't stand but when it was finally over you were amazed at how upset you were that it was finished.

I turned on the controls to start the belt moving and my heart began to pound in my chest with anticipation. I mounted the treadmill and began to increase my speed and started to jog. 1 minute went by and no pain, 3 minutes no pain, 5 minutes went by and I had to stop because I was tired but not because of any pain!! I Did Not Have Any Pain at All, Praise the Lord,

Praise The Lord!!! I felt so blessed so alive and so powerful and so thankful that God had allowed me to experience pain free running again. What a great God we serve! What a mighty God we serve! I felt so good but I also felt so humble and ready to do whatever God would tell me to do. He had just blessed me so much. I wanted to do whatever he asked me to do.

From that day I started running at least five days per week. I would increase my running by one minute more every other day until I was able to run 30 to 40 minutes at a time. It was not easy, as a matter of fact it was a great struggle but just thinking about the fact that I was not able to run for over 3 years was incentive enough to make me push myself. I felt like a young man again as if I had been remade and rejuvenated. The weight started to come off slowly but surely about 2 pounds a week and that really felt great. After I lost about 17 pounds it started to become a little harder to lose but I was just thankful for the fact that I lost what I did & I did not have any more pain.

What a miraculous thing God has done for me. The old people use to say that the Lord had brought them from a mighty long way and I heard them but I did not understand what they meant. It is one thing to hear something and intellectualize it. To know what they meant with your mind and to understand it in your mind, but when you experience something and you understand it in your heart that puts it on a whole different level of revelation and understanding. My appreciation for what had happened was much greater and on a much deeper level than it ever would've been if I had not experienced it.

I know that God is very efficient and that he does not waste anything especially not a great opportunity such as this. To have someone that is so in love with him and has been so humbled and has been made so compliant that I am truly willing to do whatever it is he will assign me to do and do it to the best of my ability without any complaints or questions. All I want the Lord to do is to tell me my mission and to provide the direction and leadership I need to achieve it and I will go, and I will do it. Please Speak Lord, Speak.

Often times in our quest to hear from God and to receive his revelation we tried to assist or encourage him to hurry up and provide us with the direction, guidance and leadership that only he can provide. It can be frustrating to be sitting there like a cocked gun just waiting to be discharged, waiting to be fired; waiting to explode into the mission and destiny that God has waiting for us. It is during these times when one must understand that God knows the precise time and the exact moment that we are ready to be released into that destiny with maximum effectiveness.

Just as a master baker knows that if he does not allow the cake too bake long enough it won't be done or if it takes too long it will be burnt and ruined. But just at the right precise time if he removes the cake from the oven he will achieve the desired results. As the master creator of our lives God has a precise exact time that he wants to release us into our true destiny and we must trust and wait on him. God will make sure that we are ready to be released before he will release us.

If you are ready to go and God has not moved yet just wait, I said wait on the Lord. He may not come when you want him, but he is always right on time.

Chapter 14

A Little Bit Goes a Long Way

"For bodily exercise profiteth little: but godliness is profitable unto all things, having promised of the life that now is, and of that which is to come." 1st.Timothy 4:8

When one looks at this verse it seems to suggest that bodily exercises is not worth much, that it will only profit us a little. On the other hand godliness will profit us in every possible way, while we are living this life and after when we pass on and go to heaven the verse continues. So I guess that all of us can forget about doing any physical activity, or becoming involved in any workout classes or doing anything physical. Everyone who reads this verse can now throw away their workout shoes, burn up all their sweat suits and workout clothes and retire to the buffets and restaurants. We can now throw away all of our treadmills and body by Jake equipment, turn on the TV and lie on the couch and just become a Couch Potato Baby! Bodily exercise does not benefit us at all right? Let's ask a few people what they think.

If we were to ask Billy Blanks if exercise profited him any I'm sure he would tell us that he has a program that will get you in great shape but he also generated more than $36 million from the sale of his tae bo products in just the first year. Now if you don't think that's profitable or beneficial Billy needs to kick some sense into you with one of his tae bo kicks. Or what about

Lebron James, he said that he had to work so hard and do lots of physical exercise to develop his game and take it to its present level, but he was rewarded with a $90 million endorsement deal and a $60 million basketball contract. I think that was pretty beneficial and profitable. What if we would ask Beyoncé if bodily exercise profited her? She would tell us that she runs, dances and lifts weights in order to be the kind of physical presence that she is. She also says working out helps her singing. Because of her physical presence and her singing talent she is able to have recording and movie contracts that are worth millions of dollars. So bodily exercise has definitely been profitable to her.

So why would Paul, an extremely highly educated and renowned thinker make a statement that bodily exercise profits us very little? What Paul is doing is comparing the amount of time during our lives that we will be able to benefit from bodily or physical things and the amount of time that we will be able to benefit from Godly or spiritual things. The only time we will be able to benefit from physical things is when we are living in our physical bodies. But we can benefit from Godly things while we are in this physical body but once we leave our physical body we can still benefit from Godly things in our eternal bodies.

Paul is saying that the amount of time that we spend in our physical bodies is very small compared to the amount of time that we will spend in our eternal bodies. If we were to compare the amount of time that we will spend in our physical bodies to the amount of time that we are going to spend in our eternal bodies it would be like comparing one drop of water (the time spent in our physical bodies) to all of the other bodies of water in the world (the time spent in our eternal bodies). Quite simply what Paul is saying is this; bodily exercise will only profit us while we are living in our bodies. That the only time bodily exercise will profit us is while we are living. If you are dead bodily exercise will not profit you! If you are dead, bodily exercise will not profit you! If you are dead reading this book ain't going to help you much either!!

However if we are alive, bodily exercise will profit us a lot. I just have one question to ask you, are you dead or are you alive?

Would all the dead people who are reading this book please raise your hands? Now would all the people that are alive who are reading this book please raise your hands? It seems to me that most of the people reading this book are alive and would benefit from bodily exercise. However there was one guy out there who didn't raise his hand for either group. But since I can see him he must be alive.

So I guess we better go get our workout shoes back, put the fire out on our sweat suits, go get our treadmills and body by Jake equipment and ease up on the buffets and restaurants and get ready to do some exercise.

My wife Kathy has heard me say many times too many people, either you will exercise before the doctor tells you or after the doctor tells you but you will exercise. But why is it so necessary for us to exercise? Have you ever noticed if you have a job where you're sitting all day? Your muscles are tight, you're back and your shoulders ache and you may have a headache and you haven't even done anything physical. Now think about how your body feels after a workout. Your muscles are warm and flexible; your heart is pounding pumping oxygen rich blood to your muscles to energize them. You feel alive, vibrant, proud of yourself and confident that you can take on the world and win. You feel much different don't you, why? Because our bodies were made to move around not to sit around!! We need to move our bodies!!!

But there are also other benefits to working out and I know you want to know what they are and I'm going to tell you. Weight loss, more energy, reduced stress; increase bone density, better sleep, stronger heart and lungs, greater interests and desire in our husband or wife are some of the benefits we receive from working out. We can also feel good about the fact that we are setting a good example for our children and grandchildren. We now have an epidemic of childhood obesity and I bet the fact that we have so many overweight adults has something to do with that. There is an old saying, "some things are more often caught then taught". Children watch us and see what we do and imitate us even when we try to tell them to do what we say and not what we do. Maybe we ought to take it upon ourselves to sacrifice and loose weight and get in shape for our children.

Then maybe they would see our example and began to participate in more physical activity themselves. One of the amazing things I've noticed about my six grandchildren is if I sit around and let them sit around too they will do it all day long. But if I get out the football or the basketball and start throwing or shooting them around I noticed that they will get out there and start having fun throwing or shooting the ball and eventually they will have a ball. One of things that we should hate the most is to hear the words "I am bored" coming out of our children or grandchildren's mouths.

How can they be bored when they are not straight A students? How can they be bored when they are not great athletes? How can they be bored when they are not in the best physical condition that they can get in? How can they be bored when they are not doing any voluntary charity work? How can they be bored when they are not employed? Oh yeah, how can they be bored when their room and their house is not at least a little bit clean?

We need to start training our children on how to become more giving and productive and how to use their time in more worthwhile and beneficial ways. If your children or grandchildren don't know everything that there is to know, then it would behoove them to turn off the cell phone, the iPod, the computer, the TV, the Blackberry and any other electronic appliance, (unless they are using them for educational purposes) and pick up an old-fashioned book and just sit down and do something unusual, be quiet and read the book. Or how about going to the YMCA, the boys club or other organization or walking around your neighborhood and getting a little exercise. The only reason why a person is bored is because they're not doing anything that is challenging to them. Get up Get out and Do Something!

What kind of exercise program should we do? The most important thing to do before starting any excise program is to go talk to our primary care physician to make sure we are able to participate in an exercise program. After we have done that and we have been given a clean bill of health to participate we should select a program that incorporates cardiovascular fitness to help us burn fat and maintain a healthy weight. We also need a strength-building component to help us stay strong and provide shape for our bodies.

What is the best cardiovascular exercise to do? The best cardiovascular exercise for us to do is one that is safe and will help us reach our fitness goals. The exercise should engage our large muscles (legs, hips, shoulders, abdomen, back and chest) when we do it. There are many different ones that a person can do that will engage these muscles. One of the most effective is walking and this is a very inexpensive yet effective form of exercise. If we were to start now, today and walk just one minute that would be a great start. If we were to add one minute every week, in 30 weeks we would have a 30-minute cardiovascular program. If we were to add one minute a week for 52 weeks we would almost be up to an hour and that would be fantastic. I'm getting excited just talking about this simple and effective way to construct a great workout program.

If we were to add a little hand weights while we were walking we would now have a muscle-building component in our program. And if we were to increase our pace while carrying the weights we could really get a great workout. To strengthen our leg muscles we could place a chair against the wall and hold on to the back of the chair and do squats 3-5 reps for 2 sets. Next we could place our hands on the wall and do push aways from the wall 3-5 reps for 2 sets for upper body strength. But there are many different exercise programs that we can do, just choose one so we can do something! Remember a little bit goes a long way!

I'm not saying that we should not have entertainment opportunities and times to just relax and forget about the cares of the day and have fun. My wife Kathy and I take 2 cruises per year to relax and enjoy ourselves. We have a great travel agency run by Julie G.; her agency is called "Dr. Tripp Travel". She puts together vacation packages that are just what the doctor ordered. When you finish one of her vacations you feel great! I can't wait for the next one. We all must have time to relax and go on vacation. It helps you to come alive.

But we cannot make the pursuit of fun become our only motive for living. If we are pursuing fun at the expense of work and excellence then that is something that we must improve on in order to become the best that we can become. We only have so many hours in the day, in the week, in the month and in the year, and we can never get that minute or hour that just passed back again. How we are using our time now is going to determine what we will become later. If we are wasting our time now it is going to add up to a wasted life later.

We are worth too much and we are much too valuable to waste our time on things that will not help us expose and develop the great value that is inside of all of us. We need to decide today, right now, this very moment, this very second that we will use our time, our talents and everything that we have too become the best that we can become. When we do this we will have the real true joy and happiness that comes from giving our best first and accomplishing the most we could with what we have. You will begin to have those moments known as those, "man I can't believe I was able to do that" moments. Or one of those, "I don't know how I did it but I knew I had to do it" moments! Let's make a commitment and a pledge to God and to ourselves to start giving Our Best Efforts First, right now because we are worth it! We are worth it! We are worth it!

It was Christmas night and I was awakened from my sleep when I heard a noise coming from the kitchen; it was very subtle as if there was someone sneaking around in there. I rose from the bed with cat like quickness and stealth. I picked up my Glock nine and deftly grabbed my machete and hurriedly glanced at the clock that now read 1:00 a.m. I tiptoed into the already lit kitchen. As I entered the kitchen I noticed that there were about five of them sitting at the table and about three others standing at various points in the room. As I lowered my Glock and took aim I noticed that these were some of the most unusual looking "things" I had ever seen. They all looked like humans but they were covered with red skin, 2, 3-inch long curved horns sticking out of their heads, a foot long tail and long claw like nails.

As I slowly squeezed the trigger I didn't notice that there were two more of them that had snuck up on each side of me and as I squeezed the trigger they hit my arm causing me to miss my target and knocking the gun out of my hand. Before I knew it all of them were attacking me and trying to throw me to the floor of my kitchen. I fought them off but there seemed to be about a dozen of them and after about an hour they finally were able to subdue me.

If only I wouldn't have eaten all that holiday food, I wouldn't feel so sluggish right now. I should have had a <u>V8!! I'd be whopping on their red behinds right now if I had my V8!!</u> They sat me down at the table and tied me to a chair. The leader told me that he was the devil and that the other creatures were his demons. They began to place in front of me all of the foods from our holiday dinner. Macaroni and cheese that is so good that it will knock you to your knees. Sweet potato pie that will make you cry, glazed ham, candied yams, potato salad, mashed potatoes and gravy, biscuits, cornbread, fried chicken, meatloaf, stewed tomatoes, green beans and collard greens.

My wife Kathy is the greatest cook in the world; hands down no one is even close. The first six months of our marriage I gained 15 pounds; we had to start eating out just so I could lose weight. I knew the food would be tasty but I was full and I did not want to eat anything else right now. So I told the devil and his little demon looking friends thank you but I'm not hungry right now and I do not want anything to eat. To my surprise the demons grabbed my head, and the devil forced open my mouth and begin stuffing the various foods in my mouth.

I didn't want to eat but they made me do it. They were just stuffing my mouth and making me eat. The devil kept on stuffing the food in my mouth over and over again. Macaroni and cheese, potato salad, ham, candy yams, fried chicken and mashed potatoes and gravy, the devil kept stuffing it in my mouth over and over again. After awhile I just stopped fighting and started to eat the food and tried to enjoy it. After all the food was delicious and there were so many of them and I was so tired that I just stopped fighting and ate the food. I didn't want to eat all that food but the devil made me do it! That's right the devil made me do it!

> *"For we wrestle not against flesh and blood, but against principalities, against powers, against the rulers of the darkness of this world, against spiritual wickedness in high places." (Ephesians 6: 12)*

Obviously there was no devil or demons in my kitchen that woke me up and forced me to eat that extra late night meal. However, the battle that we fight in our minds and our attempt to resist the temptations of the devil is all too real. It is just as tough to engage in spiritual warfare with the devils in our minds, as it is to fight anyone else in the world that exists outside our heads! We are in a constant battle, 24 hours a day with the devil and his demons and it seems that the rulers of the darkness have greater strength, power and influence at night.

Why do we find ourselves in a fight to resist the temptations of the devil and his demons especially at nighttime or in the early morning? The reason why it is hard for us to resist is because the devil and his demons are the rulers of the night. It's as if we are trying to win the battle fighting their game and playing on their field at the best time for them & not us. When we are awake that late at night or that early in the morning, we are tired and weaker and we are not at our strongest or best and are easily influenced or tempted. If we also add some alcohol or drugs into the equation we are also functioning at a diminished capacity of being confused and not thinking clearly.

I wish I had a dollar for every time I've heard someone say if I had not been drinking I would not have done this thing or that thing. Or if I had not been so a high on this drug or that drug I would not have done that. Then there are the times when we read about the multi-car accidents where there is alcohol and drugs involved either late at night or early in the morning. That is why it is so important for us to make a pact with God and ourselves that we are going to have a personal curfew and be in the bed & asleep at a reasonable hour. That way we can get the kind of rest that we need and we won't be out fighting the devil and his demons in our kitchen, on his terms and at his time.

If we make these little, tiny, minute, miniscule and small changes in our attitudes toward exercise and eating, we will be amazed at how quickly we can make our health, our physical fitness and the quality of our life so much better. I believe that no matter who you are or how young or old you may be, or how rich or poor you may be no matter what your situation in life is, if you will apply these principles to your life, I'm sure that you're going to have a major breakthrough in your life. I'm just so happy and excited for you. Just remember a little bit goes a long way!

Dr. M.D. Brown, 1st. note: If we don't eat anything after 8:00 p.m. until breakfast time the next day, we will be surprise how much more weight we can lose!!

Chapter 15

Everyone Catches & Goes Through Hell Sometimes!

"And we know that all things work together for good to them that love God, to them who are the called according to his purpose."(Romans 8:28)

Everyone catches some hell in their lives or goes through hell sometimes. On their job, and in their relationships, in their marriage, and their family lives or the many other situations that we are involved in during our lifetime. What we must endeavor to do is while we are catching hell we must not hold on to it. We must learn to let it go. While we are going through hell we must make sure that we keep on going and that we do not stop!" The premise I am establishing is that we all are going to go through troubles and difficult times in our lives but we must not get stuck or stop when going through those tough and difficult times. We must go ahead and go through those times without stopping. We must get to the other side of our trials & tribulations.

We all are going to catch some hell in our lives but we can make a choice to hold on to that hell or let that hell go. There are times when we will have horrible situations come up in our lives that if we stop and dwell on those situations, they can cause us to become so obsessed with them that we will not have time for anything else. They can cause us to drop right out of our normal routine and place in society and totally shut down and become unable to function normally. We can be catching so much hell that the only way for us to cope, if we hold on to it is to go temporarily or permanently insane. Some things that we face and encounter can literally disturb us so much that we can lose our minds. Sometimes we can receive so much bad news and in such a short period of time that if it was not for our faith in Jesus and our belief that God would make it all right we would go completely cuckoo and crazy.

Even though it may seem like things are so bad and dark sometimes and that there is no way for them to be straightened out or get brighter. I want you to think about Romans 8: 28, because God will make all the things that we could possibly go through work together for our good. He has a purpose for us and sometimes we have to go through some things in order for him to prepare us to be able to step into our purpose. You see God understood that in order for us to be ready to run a marathon we must first go through the pain and training of running a mile. God must condition us by putting us through things so that we're able to handle even bigger things and greater challenges. If we can trust him in the little things and in the preliminary stages of our lives, we will know that we can trust him in the bigger and better parts of our lives.

That is exactly what happened in my wife Kathy's life. As a young girl she was faced with one tragedy after another and it appeared as if they would never cease. She comes from a very close and large family of 10 children who loved each other very much. There were eight sisters and 2 brothers. The sister whom Kathy was closest to was Cynthia. They went everywhere together and really had fun with each other. Cynthia became very sick and had to be taken to the hospital. Even though her sister was in a hospital about 60 miles away in another city, Kathy and her mother would go visit her almost every day. Her sister had a lengthy illness that culminated in her passing away. Kathy was 15 and Cynthia was 14 at the time of her departure from this life. The loss devastated Kathy and left her asking God why did he have to take her sister. She questioned God but she did not doubt him or turn her back on God but her young, tender mind could not understand it at that time. Little did she know that this was just the beginning of the sorrows for her family.

One day Kathy's father was not feeling well and the next thing the family knew, he had a stroke that caused him to be hospitalized. He was in the hospital for about two months and was brought home in a hospital bed still not fully recovered. The family was very concerned but her mother worked with him diligently and helped him to achieve an almost total recovery. But from that point on her father never worked again.

One of her sisters lived in Chicago in a high-rise apartment. One day while her sister's daughter Cindy was playing by an open window, somehow Cindy fell out and plunged to her death! Little Cindy was only three years old. Why did such a young and innocent child have to die such a tragic and sudden death Kathy wondered? How could Kathy make any sense out of this event? What was the purpose for this?

A few years later another tragedy struck the family. Kathy's sister Belinda was discovered in her car, dead. Somehow her car had caught fire and she had died from smoke inhalation. To make things worse this occurred on her sister's birthday. The remaining family members were devastated and this was another great blow for Kathy and she didn't know how she would make it but somehow she did. In the new King James Version of the Bible we find these words of comfort in *Psalms 18:5 & 6: "The sorrows of Sheol surrounded me; The snares of death confronted me. In my distress I call upon the Lord, And cried out to my God; He heard my voice from His temple, And my cry came before Him, even to his ears."*

Sometimes when we're going through a period of sorrow and despair, it's just good to know that God is there and that he hears our prayers and our cares and that he cares. Maybe that's a good example for us to use when we are comforting someone who is going through their particular hell or sorrows. If we can just be there to listen and not to condemn or judge but just listen. Because sometimes life does not make sense and we need to know someone is there to hear our cries and is listening.

A few months later her father fell into another coma and was unable to recover and passed away. This Horrific Tragedy Occurred Just Three Days Before Christmas of That Year! Her sister had just passed away in August and now this!! Kathy said that this turned out to be an even greater blow for her to adjust to then the loss of her sisters and her niece. She said watching her mother and how she was able to cope with the losses and keep the family together helped her to keep going. What else can go wrong?

She would help her mother during this time and developed a bond with her. Kathy often asked her mother how she was able to handle all of the losses and cope with them, as well as she was able to. Her mother explained to her that you will be amazed at what you can handle if you have to. God will always make a way for you if you just believe and trust in him. Her mother said the Lord works in mysterious ways his wonders to perform. Kathy saw her mother's faith and belief in God and even though she didn't understand it at the time, or the reason why, she felt a lot better and a bit stronger.

Isn't it amazing what mothers can do, how they can put our minds at ease and make us feel better just by saying a couple of words. How they can stroke our brows and that simple caress, that little touch can make us feel so much better. Mothers can make us feel secure, safe and loved with just a touch. I want all the mothers to know that you're God's special agents here on earth and your mission as mothers is such a very important and special one. Don't let anyone tell you that you are not important. Don't let anyone tell you that you are not vital. Don't let anyone tell you that you don't make a difference. All you mothers are very very special. And you mothers don't get to hear that enough. On behalf of all of us who have mothers and don't tell them enough that we love them and just how special you mothers are, I want to say we love you and we thank you for all that you do. What a difference you mothers make in our lives. Thank you, Thank you, Thank you.

Several years later Kathy's mother had jokingly told Kathy that she had gotten lost going home and that it took her a little while to remember how to get back home but eventually she did. This happened to her on several occasions and Kathy began to observe her a little closer. She took her mother to the doctor for an examination and it was discovered that she was in the early stages of Alzheimer's disease. One of Kathy's sisters Dorothy, who was probably the best nurse that you could be under the care of, talked with the family about the disease.

The prognosis was that the disease could be treated with various medications in a hope to stop its progress but that it would be best for her mother not to live alone. Kathy's youngest sister Robin decided that she and her son Miles would move back home and stay with her mother. A couple years later Robin moved them into her dream home and everything seemed to be going very well. Robin was a very good Christian lady that loved the Lord. She also was a highly respected professional in the field of social work. She had a great position and her services were highly sought after on a contract basis. Robin's life is going great and everything seemed to be perfect, everything seemed to be falling in place. Everything seemed too good to be true. How many of you out there know that when everything seems to be too good to be true that that's when you better watch out because all Hell is about ready to break loose!!

Robin called Kathy and told her that she was not feeling well, that she was sick. This went on for about two years and her health began to deteriorate over this period of time. She would have periods of time where she would vomit on several occasions, once she even vomited blood. When Kathy was transporting her to and from the dr., Kathy would have to stop the car so that Robin could vomit. A couple of times Robin went into a catatonic stupor that rendered her motionless and caused her to be hospitalized. She would stay in this state until she received medical assistance. As Robin's condition worsened, it was discovered that she needed to have a liver transplant, which was a very serious operation.

Through all of this Kathy was encouraging her and helping her with her mother, her son and her other obligations. To Kathy's surprise she had the strength, the intestinal fortitude and the desire to help. It was during this time that she realized what God had been preparing her to do with those past situations and past tragedies. They helped her to be able to handle the things that she was encountering now. She still didn't understand why those things had happened to the people that they had happened to; maybe God would reveal that to her later. But Kathy knew that going through it had made her stronger and more capable of functioning in situations such as these.

Everyone was optimistic, hopeful and prayed up; we all believed that everything would be okay. Robin was a good Christian woman that read her Bible and prayed everyday so we knew that God was on our side. Robin had the surgery but did not survive and She Died in the hospital. What another horrible calamity for the family. It was as if the hits just kept on coming, blow after blow after blow. It seemed like sometimes if we didn't receive bad news there was not any news at all! Amen.

Besides Robin's death there were other issues to deal with. Who was going to care for her son? Who would provide care for her mother with Alzheimer's? Who would handle the arraignments for her funeral and all the other problems that arise when someone passes away? Kathy with help from her other sisters, Dorothy, Gladys, Ivra, and Carol, her special friend Carmen, her daughter Starla and Miles handled these duties. Everyone did a great job taking care of their responsibilities and their obligations. One would think that this was enough tragedy for one family to face in such a short period of time but hold on there is more coming.

We had Robin's son Miles come and live with our family during this time. One day he called Kathy from school, complaining that he did not feel well and was sick. She went to pick him up from the school, when she went in to sign him out, Miles had to go back to the office to get his bookbag that he had forgotten. As he was returning, Kathy saw him falling, as if in slow motion. She went over to him and saw that he was still breathing but semi-conscious. She had the attendant called 911 and Miles was taken to the hospital and was diagnosed with having kidneys failure. Kathy's daughter Starla met them at the hospital and was very helpful to Miles and assisted him greatly during his emergency room and hospital stay.

Miles was later placed on dialysis for almost 18 months and Kathy took him to most of those appointments with help from Robin's friend Carmen. It was determined that he would have to have a kidney transplant because his kidneys had completely failed. More bad news and especially in view of the fact that his mother had died during a transplant operation! Kathy had to encourage Miles to believe that God would make it all right even though she was still grieving her sister passing.

She would often read Philippians 4:19 for strength which reads: *But my God shall supply all your need according to his riches in glory by Christ Jesus.* (Philippians 4:19) Kathy realized that if she relied upon her own strength and understanding that she would probably go out of her mind, but thank God that he was meeting her needs every step of the way. When she needed help to handle the tragedy of someone's death, God provided that help. When she needed help at the hospital, God provided that help. When she needed help to encourage someone, God gave her the words to say. Every time that she needed some help having any of her needs met, God was always there and available to meet her needs!

And I'm here to encourage you today, to let you know that just as God was there to meet Kathy's needs he will be there to meet yours also. All you have to do is make Jesus Christ the Savior and Lord of your life and you will have access to the one and only true God that can really do something for you and is able to meet every need that you have. Amen-Amen-Amen!! John 14:6 reads:

Jesus saith unto him, I am the way, the truth, and the life: no man, cometh unto the Father, but by me. The only way for us to have a way to reach God, to know the truth and to have a real life is through his son Jesus Christ. If you follow anybody else you're headed in the wrong direction and you will be lost.

Miles had the kidney transplant and it was a tremendous success. His doctors said that they had not seen a patient recover as quickly as he did before. He was truly blessed and he was very thankful. He was able to finish high school and graduated with his class and he is now attending college and doing very well. God can make a difference in your life can't he? Kathy was now feeling pretty good about the way that Miles had come out of his transplant and she was coping with her grief from her sister's death a lot better. It seemed as if things were starting to turn around and get better but we all know when everything looks like it's getting better, you better watch out!

Kathy and her sister Dorothy, who is a nurse, were on the telephone just having girl talk and Dorothy matter-of-factly told Kathy that she had been a little dizzy lately but she just dismissed it as being overworked from the two positions which she was working and that she was going to get some rest and she knew she would be feeling better. About two months later, after she had returned from vacation, Dorothy complained that she was still having dizzy spells and that her vision in her right eye had gotten blurry. She went in for a checkup about three months later and it was discovered that she had spots on her brain that showed she had brain cancer. Dorothy had called Kathy and told her that she was very afraid. Kathy took a week off and went to visit her and encourage her. Dorothy started treatment but in about four weeks her cancer had spread and she was only given a little while to live. Many people had been praying for her but Dorothy did not recover.

Kathy went back to Chicago to spend some time with Dorothy but Dorothy had slipped into a coma and did not come out of it. Sometimes God works in mysterious ways his wonders to perform Kathy said. Through all of this Kathy had learned that even though you're going through hell, life must still go on and there must be someone who can help others get through that hell. Because there is always going to be some hell in every bodies life, but if you have Faith in God he will bring you through. The book of Job explains this in 14th chapter verse 1: *"Man that is born of a woman is of few days and full of trouble."* We will not live long, relatively speaking, and the few days that we will live are going to be full of trouble. Thank God he had prepared those people like Kathy who can help us make it through.

Those of you who do not have anyone in your family that has that special talent to care and have compassion, yet are able to function and pull it together. During those tragic times when we all need someone to take control and get done the things that need to be done in order for life to go on. I am praying for you that someone will step forward in your family and accept that role. You may be the one who can do it. Life has so many hellish moments that we all need someone who can fill that role and help keep our families going.

To all of you who have suffered loss or are going through loss right now, I want you to know that you are in our hearts and in our prayers and that we love you and are concerned about you. May the Lord provide you with the comfort and peace that only he can give and may joy and happiness follow you for the rest of your days.

But I also want you to remember this as long as you may live:

If you are catching hell in your life don't hold it, you must throw it down, you must throw it down, you must throw down, throw it down, throw down! And if you're going through hell you must not stop, you must keep going, keep going, keep going, keep going! "

Chapter 16

You Can Fool Some People But You Can't Fool Mom!

"What! Know ye not that your body is the temple of the Holy Ghost which is in you, which you have of God, and ye are not your own? For ye are bought with a price: therefore glorify God in your body, and in your spirit, which are God's."(1st. Corinthians 6:19 & 20)

Paul is explaining to every Christian that our bodies are the dwelling places of God or the houses of God. What he means is that the third person of the trinity, the Holy Spirit, resides in us and can lead, direct and guide us from that position. We must be willing to let the Holy Spirit have control, but he is a gentleman; he will not force himself on us and make us do something that we don't want to do. Every Christian represents God's house and as such, we are to glorify or make God look good, both in our physical appearance and in the way we behave and live.

Paul is also saying that as Christians our bodies are not our own and that they have been loaned to us by God. God is our landlord; he is the one that we rent this body from. He is the one that has allowed us the privilege of living in this fantastic mechanism known as the human body. We are a walking, talking, breathing, seeing, feeling and thinking miracle! This thing we call the human body is really something very, very, very special. There is not another machine anywhere that can do what this human body can do. It does not matter how much money you may have; you cannot buy another brand-new human body! Every human being is so special that we are priceless.

What if God were to act like your mom and he were to look at our bodies, what would he say? And what would he do? Would he look at us and say that we had enhanced his property and have added value to his property? Would he tell you, well done my good and faithful servant? You know I just love what you've done with your ab muscles, they are so hard and lean and flat. And your obliques are so trim and fat-free, how'd you get them like that? I just love what you've done with your gluteus maximus it's so tight, round and firm. Normally those can be such a problem but you seem to have it all under control!

Or would God-mom look at us and say what have you done to my property? Looks like you let yourself go, what happened to you? I've been trying to check out your stomach muscles but with all that fat you have around them I can't even see them. Every time you walk your gluteus maximus looks like 2 dogs fighting in a bag. And those fat thighs are not really necessary are they? If you don't get it together you're going to end up destroying this house! If you don't think you'll do it, you need to read these verses in 1st. Corinthians 3: 16 & 17: *"Know ye not that ye are the temple of God, and that the spirit of God dwelleth in you? If any man defile the temple of God, him shall God destroy; for the temple of God is holy, which temple ye are."* God-mom would say "I love you but you better get this place straightened up!"

This is one verse that really causes me much personal pain and grief. Why? Because I have seen so many people who have had to suffer because of it. The literal meaning of the verse is that you cannot defile the church that is built upon Jesus Christ. If one would do that then God shall destroy him. But the allegory meaning could be this; since we are the temple or the dwelling place of God, if someone were to defile "us", would God then destroy them? Now if we were guilty of causing that defilement ourselves, could we be in danger of being destroyed by God? In other words, if we did things to hurt our own bodies or our own health would we be guilty of defiling the temple of God?

If we were to conclude that this is true then it would be possible for us to be guilty of causing our own destruction. Indulging in behaviors such as drug abuse, illicit sexual activity, alcohol abuse, eating disorders, over working, over exercising or under exercise and other self-destructive behaviors. This could explain why so many people have died at such young ages from diseases such as sugar diabetes, high blood pressure, heart disease, cancers, obesity, strokes, cirrhosis of the liver and infectious diseases. Because they defiled their bodies God destroyed them or God allowed the natural progression of these self-destructive tendencies to take their course and culminate in their deaths.

What a sobering thought if this is true, but we can do something about this to change it. I would like to tell you about some individuals whom I knew and about some of the sad stories associated with them that fit into this category. I want you to know that I'm not telling you these things to make you feel bad or to frighten you but I'm telling you these things in an effort to heighten your awareness and to help you to avoid these catastrophes. I want you to say something right now! Dr. M. D. Brown, 1st. is not here to hurt you he's here to help you. I believe that God will bless me with the words that will reach you because I do not want anyone to experience the level of pain or hurt that my family and I have experienced.

The telephone rang on 4/7/'93 at about 7 a.m. Before I answered it I knew something was wrong. We all know how it is when one of those calls comes in that before we answer it we know it's baaaad news. It was my sister Violet and she told me that my mother and father were preparing to take my older brother Alonzo to the hospital because he had complained of chest pains. She told me that he had a heart attack in the back of their van and that they were proceeding to take him to the hospital as we were speaking. I told her I would be there shortly. I hung up, quickly got dressed and headed for the hospital that my parents were taking my brother to. But the Holy Spirit told me to go in a different direction.

Instead of going to the hospital I went to the nearest fire station and as I knocked on the fire station's door I noticed some clothing in front of the big overhead door. It was my brother's coat and shirt and I observed that they had been cut off of him by the way they were torn and tattered. There was no one at the fire station so as I picked up his clothing I also saw medical supplies scattered about which must have been used to administer to him while he was there. I proceeded to go to the hospital and as I got there, I was informed that the emergency squad had just brought him in. My parents were just going into the family room and I met them there and was brought up to date on what had happened. I also tried to provide whatever comfort I could to them.

One of the doctors came in and spoke with us briefly and said that one of us could go back and be with Alonzo in the E.R. while they worked on him. Our mother asked me to go back and told me to make sure that I pinched the inside of his lip because she read somewhere that if a person has a heart attack you pinch their lip and they'll recover. I was thinking to myself if my mother said to try it then I'll try it, the bumps went away didn't they!

I went back and watched as the team shocked his heart, injecting him with various medications and assisted his breathing. I went in with the belief that he was going to be all right and that God would deliver him. I inched close to his head and while I was praying in his ear I moved my hand next to his lip and with my fingers was able to pinch his lip. Unfortunately this did not work the first time so I tried it three more times but again it was unsuccessful. As time passed it was apparent that we would not be successful in reviving my brother. I was praying and asking God not to let him die, to intervene and help the doctors bring him back.

The doctor looked at me and told me there was nothing more that the team could do for him. I asked them not to stop but to give him a little more time. They worked on him for 10 more minutes and I was praying furiously hoping that God would bring him back. But the team was unsuccessful and the doctor told me that my brother's heart attack was so severe that it was as if his heart had exploded in his chest! The doctor said that with my brother carrying so much extra weight that it was just a matter of time before this was going to happen. He told the team to stop, he pronounced the time of death and my oldest brother departed this life just that quickly and suddenly.

If you've ever seen someone die then you know that feeling, that knawing, that sick nauseating feeling you get in the pit of your stomach. Well when you watch a loved one die you multiply that by 10 and then you add unto that the abrupt shock, the hopelessness, and the sudden finality of it all that leaves you with a sadness and pain that is hard to describe. Then you couple that with the fact that you must be the one who brings this horrible devastating news to your family members, and especially to his and your mother!

As I went back to the family room preparing myself for the questions and for the family prayer, suppressing my grief and pain preparing to provide the needed counseling and comfort my family members would need. As a pastor and a counselor one is trained to divorce oneself from the emotional aspects of an event, of a tragedy and be the voice of strength, faith, confidence and hope.

When I entered the room to face the expectant and hopeful looks of my family, I went to our mother first. I hugged her and explained to her that the doctors had worked hard and put forth their best efforts possible to revive Alonzo. I told her that I had pinched his lip repeatedly and had prayed for him ferociously, but all our best efforts were unfruitful and that now our brother and her son was with the Lord. He was not suffering any more pain and that he was resting in the arms of God and enjoying all the joys of living in heaven. As expected everyone began crying and my mother became hysterical, crying my baby, my baby, my baby, my baby is gone and running up and down in the parking lot. After about a half an hour we finally got her calmed down and was able to get her back inside and have the family prayer.

All the family went to the room that our brother and our mother's son was in and said our goodbyes. We prayed again and we could really feel the spirit in the room as we thanked God for the amount of time that we were blessed to have had our brother and our mother's son. But you know there was a sadness and a void that we had never experienced before. This was the first time since I had been living that my oldest brother was not living. It was also the first time that our mother had lost a child. What a terrible thing for any mother to have to experience, the death of her first born child. Especially when the death of her child occurred right in front of her eyes as she was attempting to get him some help.

My mother began to review the course of events of the day stating that my father and she were transporting her son to the hospital when he had a heart attack in the back of their van. They took him to the fire station near the house and the paramedics cut his coat and shirt off and began CPR and defibrillation on him. They got a slight pulse, loaded him up in the ambulance and transported him to the hospital. She said she thought he had a chance as she rode in the back of the ambulance with her son as the paramedics worked on her son. They wouldn't allow her to go back to the room that they had taken her son to, to work on him. At the hospital I had faith in God to make my son okay. That's when you showed up, Mark and I knew he'd be okay.

Then our mother began to cry saying over and over again I just can't believe this has happened, I just can't believe this has happened.

The pain, the helplessness, the hurt, the hopelessness, the confusion and the emptiness that began to encompass our family was almost overwhelming. I thought of all the times that I had comforted other people with what I thought were words of comfort and hope, feeling as if I had done something significant; realizing now that there are no words that can bring my mother's son back or ease the pain that she feels in her heart for this tragic loss. My mother would say that no mother should have to experience the loss of her child and that the natural order of things was for the parents to pass away first then the children. Wanting to ease the pain I thought what could I do?

The doctor's statement echoed in my mind, "with your brother carrying so much weight it was only a matter of time before this was going to happen." My brother weighted about 450 pounds; he ate about anything that he wanted to, he had been a smoker for over 25 of his 47 years and was not involved in any kind of exercise program at all. Our family history contained 8 uncles and 6 aunts that had died from heart attacks, cancers, sugar diabetes and obesity related diseases. With a lifestyle and a family history such as this, the doctor's statement made a lot of sense. But what can we do to avoid these painful outcomes such as the one my family and my mother are experiencing now?

Then my mother asked me the question, WHY DID THIS HAVE TO HAPPEN? WHY? WHY? WHY? WHY? MY MOTHER CRIED!!! WHY DID MY CHILD HAVE TO DIE? WHY?

I slowly took my mother's hands and asked her to please sit down. I calmly asked her to think of what we had talked about when my friend, we will call him "Davey Gator", had passed away at 50 years of age. "Davey" ate whatever he wanted to, he struggled with a weight problem all his life and at the time of his death he weighed over 300 pounds. He was also a smoker. I talked with Davey about his weight and health but he said, "you got to die from something but I'm going to enjoy myself before I go." He became sick with diabetes and stopped working out. He said his feet and legs were in constant pain due to his diabetes. He then had his toe amputated, then next his foot, then next his leg was amputated below the knee. Davey had high blood pressure and a heart condition, which is what he died from. My mother asked me the question why do you think he died, what happened to him?

And I told her that there are four keys that will ensure that you have a great chance of living a long life and have good health and good physical fitness. After seeing your doctor and getting a physical the four keys are:

1. Get the right kind of rest, 6-8 hours of sleep per night.
2. Eat the right kinds of foods, fruits and vegetables and lean cuts of meat, chicken, fish, ect. Limit your sweets and processed foods.
3. Exercise 30 to 40 minutes per day, walking is great but whatever exercise you do if it involves moving the big core muscles of your body it is good for you.
4. Don't put substances in your body that are bad for you: cigarettes, drugs, the wrong kinds of foods, alcohol, etc.

And my mother would always tell me that somebody needs to tell everyone about these four keys so they can have a great and healthy life.

Mom didn't understand that people do not like to be told that they need to change the lifestyle that they have become so accustomed to, even if it can save their lives. I knew what to do and I would use it for myself and my immediate associates and friends. I wasn't going to force this on anyone.

We then talked about another friend of ours that had passed away, we will call him "Smokey Car". Smoky was 47 years old when he passed away from a heart attack while he was having a dialysis treatment. Smokey had been a great athlete but he always had a weight problem and he weighed over 300 pounds most of his adult life. Smoky ate anything that he wanted without concern for his health; he really liked eating fatty meats. His exercise program had dropped off considerably and as he got older he was in poor physical condition, he had also suffered kidney failure.

I said to my mother, remember when you asked me about "Smokey Car" and what I had said I thought had happened to him? Yes she said, you said he broke your four rules to be able to live a long life. They must get the right kind of rest, eat the right kind of foods, don't put substances in their body that are bad for them, and exercise regularly. My mother said, "I had told you that someone needs to tell everyone about these rules and how important they are to help us live a long healthy life."

My mother said, "That is what happened to my son isn't it?" He was over weight, he ate badly, he was a smoker and he didn't get the rest like he should have either. She said, "I always warned him about his weight but he said he couldn't help it and that he thought I was always picking on him." I should've been more insistent and encouraging. I should have done more! Why didn't I do more, Why didn't I do more?

I told her that she had done as much as anyone could have and that there was no need for her to feel guilty or bad. I told her that I would try to tell more people about the four rules. She seemed to feel a little better. Because as a mother she said "I don't want any other mothers or families to have to experience this pain or sorrow that we are experiencing." I began to develop MDB1, Inc. for the purpose of telling people about these four rules.

I had been talking to my sister, Violet about the four rules, and she had cut down on her smoking, she had lost some weight, and she had started an exercise program. She had a job that required her to work many long hours but she was getting more rest than she had been getting. Things seemed to be improving physically for her, things were looking up. But how many of us know when things seem to be going great that's time to watch out!

The call came in on December 26, 1999, my niece Tiffany, who was Violet's daughter called and told me that Violet had been admitted to the hospital. She had not been feeling well lately and upon examination it was discovered that Violet had cancer that had spread throughout her entire body. The doctors gave her less than a month to live. It seems that Violet knew she had been sick for a while but kept on going anyway. She was always a very tough and strong person and could handle a lot of pain.

The family was devastated and the only one who knew that Violet was even a little sick was Tiffany. Our mother was extremely upset because she thought if she would've known sooner, maybe she could have done something to help. We began praying, fasting and contacting other churches to pray in a hope that a miracle could be performed by God. There is nothing that is too hard for God; he can do anything but fail!! We kept a watch at our sister's house and we all met or stayed there every day.

On January the 13th, 2000 our mother and father's daughter and our sister went home to be with the Lord. Our mother and father had stepped out to go to their home to pick up some clothing and Violet had expired in their absence. It was almost as if she did not want them to see another one of their children pass away right before their eyes so she waited until they were gone to expire. What a tragic situation, she was a good Christian woman and we knew where she was going but we just didn't expect her to be going so soon.

Violet had been doing several things to improve her health and physical fitness but sometimes things just go too far to correct. Sometimes the body just will not repair itself anymore. Sometimes the body will quit forgiving us and it will break down and stay broke down. She had made pretty good progress but it was almost a case of being too little too late for her.

After my mother and father's daughter and our sister's home going service my mother said to me, I know what happened to her now. It's those damn four rules of yours isn't it? You know what you better do don't you? Then she said to me "Mark Douglas Brown", you better tell everyone you can about your four rules so that they can live longer and healthier lives." Because I don't want any other families to have to face the kind of pain and sadness that we are facing right now. I told her that I would do that and I started to develop M,D.B.1 ministries.

Chapter 17

What Did You Say Lord? Butts, Gut's And Gray Hairs?

The telephone call came at 6:00 a.m. on October 6, 2006, it was my niece Tiffany and she told me that my mother was taken to the hospital because she was unresponsive. I told Tiffany that I would be there as soon as I got dressed. We prayed, and then I got dressed and preceded to the hospital. When I arrived at the hospital I was told that my mother, who is a diabetic, had gone into a diabetic coma due to lack of glucose to her brain and had not woke up. My mother was scheduled for several tests to determine her diagnoses & prognosis and treatment plan. Her eyes were open but she was not responding to any stimuli or movement. She had a blank look on her face. The family prayed for her and we encouraged each other and I started a week fast for her healing.

The family met with the neurologist, a very nice and upbeat man, with a tremendous bedside manner. He said that mother's brain stem was still intact which was a good sign but that she did have damage to the parts of her brain that controlled her cognition, reasoning, memory and purposeful movements. Drugs and physical therapy could potentially help her to recover. He gave us two different case scenarios; the first saw mother making a complete and total recovery being able to live a pretty much normal life. The second visualized her as needing some assistance and possibly an assisted living arrangement but that she should make a significant recovery. This is great news and we were all very optimistic about our mother's recovery. It was now October 8th 2006.

October 9, 2006, mother is moving her arms and legs very vigorously almost like someone who is running. It's difficult to keep the blanket on her body but all her movement encourages us. But she has not responded to our questions or outside stimuli purposefully, but she would briefly squeeze your hand when you would hold hers. She had not spoken to anyone and her eyes were open, but she did not look at us but passed or through us. Mother still was unable to care for herself in any way nor could she tell us what she needed. She was totally dependent upon someone else to have her needs met. We would pray for her and read scriptures from the Bible to her every day.

November 6, 2006, mother had to have a tracheotomy to assist her in breathing. She had not spoken to this point; she was still moving on her own but not purposefully and not reacting to outside stimuli. We had also brought in some of her favorite music and played it to her. My brother Richard, my niece Tiffany, my father Alonzo and myself were at the hospital or nursing home everyday. She had now been transferred to a nursing home to provide her with physical therapy as well as being able to meet her other needs.

Mother's diagnosis and her prognosis had changed quite a bit at this present time. Additional tests have been taken which have revealed that 95% of our mother's brain was destroyed and that the potential for her recovery was very minimal. As a matter of fact one doctor had said that it was only a matter of time before she would expire. We continued to pray and believe that God could provide our mother with a complete and total recovery. There were other churches and pastors praying for our mother. We knew and believed that where men have failed God has succeeded many times. This was just another time that God would show his power. We would not be discouraged in the least; we had complete and total faith in God!!

December 6, 2006, we moved mother to another nursing home because we were not happy with the care of the other one. About 20 doctors also have seen her. I can't be exactly sure because the nursing home and hospitals had other doctors see her that we didn't know about. She still has not responded to any outside stimuli, other then the occasional hand squeeze and did not demonstrate any purposeful movements. Her eyes are still open but even when she moves her head she will look through you, not at you. If you touch her forehead or wipe her face she does furrow her brow. She now has a bedsore that is being treated to prevent it from spreading. It felt so strange that we had to celebrate her birthday on 11/9/06 at the nursing home and also have thanksgiving for her there too. I didn't realize how much a loved ones sickness affects the rest of the family. I always thought that if I were to get sick or in bad health that it would only impact me and maybe my wife but our whole family has been affected.

January 6, 2007, mother had to go to the hospital because of an infection and to stabilize her blood sugar; she has been running high fevers and been susceptible to these infections for the last week. Her bedsore had gotten bigger and it was most likely the source of her infection. Because she could not feed herself, she was being fed by an abdominal pic and was not receiving the nutrition she needed to repair the bedsore, which got bigger. The bedsore was debrided and her blood sugar was stabilized.

Her diagnosis was now a condition called "persistent vegetative state". In this condition the brain is damaged in the areas responsible for consciousness, self-awareness and personality. The intact brain stem means my mother retains motor reflexes, sleep and wake cycles and the activity of her autonomic nervous system. Her involuntary movements had decreased but they were still occurring but just not as strong or as often as before. She would look in your direction sometimes but she was not aware that you were there. The prognosis was that some people recover from this condition but that the longer they are in this condition the bleaker their chances are for recovery. We celebrated

Christmas and New Year's twice; at home and with my mother at the nursing home.

February 6, 2007, mother's condition has deteriorated slightly and she is not moving around as much as she did but otherwise she's doing about the same. She has not spoken to us or acknowledged our presence since she was hospitalized back on October 6, 2006. We all sure do miss talking to her and laughing with her about something that happened during the day. We are still reading to her every day and praying with her everyday and there are whole churches that are praying for her. We still have faith and trust in God and we believe that he can do anything but fail.

March 6, 2007, mother is not moving as much as she had been and she has returned to the hospital to help stabilize her sugar levels and to get rid of another infection. The doctor was successful in stabilizing her and she was returned to the nursing facility. She's sleeping more now and appears to be very tired. She has not been able to purposely position herself in over 5 months. She has not been able to speak to us during the same period. We are still praying, the churches are still praying and we are reading and playing her favorite music to her every day. It sure would be nice to be able to hear her voice again and to hear her make jokes and laugh. Just to be able to see her smile again and tell us how proud she was of us. There is no amount of money that I would not give just to be able to have my mother restored back to her "normal self." You never realize how much you miss something so simple as a glass of water until the well runs dry. Common ordinary things can become so valuable when you do not have them anymore.

April 6, 2007, mother's condition was downgraded to "permanent vegetative state" which means that she had been in a state of permanent unawareness for six months. She was also placed on dialysis because her kidneys had failed. She is not moving much at all now and her bedsore although stabilized is quite large. The doctor says it is about 3 inches deep. The diabetes makes it difficult for the bedsore to get well. The amazing thing about her condition is that when we touch her head to wipe her face she will furrow her brow but she does not respond to pain when they put IVs or needles in her arms or stomach or legs. When we hold her hand her grip is much weaker than it had been.

The doctors asked my father in view of my mother's new diagnosis and prognosis did he want to continue her treatment and sustain her care. The doctors felt that at this juncture there was not much that they could do. The doctors said if we wanted a second opinion feel more than free to get it. My father decided to do that and we had his wife and our mother transferred to one of the leading medical facilities in our area to have her case evaluated.

A team of 15 doctors evaluated her and reviewed her case. They concluded that 95% of our mother's and my father's wife's brain had been damaged and that clinically, she met all the criteria for being classified as "unaware" or "permanent vegetative state." Her bodily functions were deteriorating and she did not have long to live naturally. The team said that artificially, with a respirator, dialysis and other machines medical science could prolong her existence indefinitely. There have been some individuals that have recovered from this condition but those occurrences were very, very rare.

In the team's opinion, the initial trauma that had occurred on October 6, 2006, when our mother and our father's wife's brain had been deprived of sugar, was so severe that she was actually brain-dead from that point forward. It has taken this long for our mother and our father's wife's body to catch up to her dead brain and die! The team stated that with this diagnosis our father could legally stop his wife's care and treatment and end her suffering.

Our father explained that he had been with this one woman for over 63 of his 80 years and that they had been through many hard times together but they made it through them all. This was just another one of those hard times and by the grace of God they would get through this one somehow. Our father said, "you experts say that some people come out of this condition; well she is going to be that one in a million, or that one in a billion that makes it." Then our father said, "my wife is not a throwaway and I am not going to throw her away. There is no way that I am going to pull the plug on her now or ever!!"

Love is a very special and unique relationship when it is done correctly and in the Lord. It unites two individuals on the physical, intellectual and spiritual level. This causes a soul tie between these two individuals that is so strong and so tight that the Bible says they become one. In the book of Genesis chapter 2 verse 24 it reads: *"Therefore shall a man leave his father and mother, and shall cleave unto his wife: and they shall be one flesh."*

Our father and mother were truly one and through the past six months of observing the things that he would do in relationship to his wife and our mother's care, he would always make one statement: "she would do the same thing for me." After cleaving with her or being one with her for all those many years, he was the best qualified to make these important and vital decisions concerning his wife's care and treatment.

What a tremendous responsibility to have the fate of your mate in your hands. If you decided that she would live then she would live. If you decided to terminate her care then she would die. If my father felt he gave his wife less than his best, he would be second-guessing and beating up on himself for the rest of his life. If one is going to err in such an important decision as this it is better to err on the side of caution. What would you do if you had to make that choice for your mate? Would you say, I finally got you where I want you now and I'm going to make you pay for all the things you did to me, Pull the Plug!! Pull the Plug!! I'm just playing; I'm just playing ok!!

Seriously what a difficult task that my father had to face and he was there everyday; he never missed a day of seeing her. He was still her protector and her eyes and her ears and her mouth and he did a fantastic job for her. The team had my father's wife and our mother returned to the nursing home. My father rode in the back of the ambulance with her holding her hand all the way.

May 6, 2007, the telephone rang and before I picked it up I knew that it was bad news; you just know down there in your "knower" when bad news comes. It was my niece Tiffany and she told me that mother had been taken to the hospital again and on the way there she had expired in the back of the ambulance. I had told her when I was out there earlier that mother really didn't look very good. It was now 9:30 p.m. and I told her I would be there momentarily. I arrived at the hospital and was taken back to the holding room where our father's wife and our mother's body was being stored. Our father, Tiffany, my brother Richard, my son Mark and I bowed and prayed for our mother. We were all extremely saddened by her departure but in a way we were relieved that our father was not forced to make the choice. God had decided for him. My father began to speak about their history together and he must have talked for about three hours and we could understand that he did not want to leave his wife anymore than we wanted to say goodbye to our mother.

Mother's condition had really deteriorated in these last days and one could tell that it would not be long before she would pass. With the sugar diabetes hard to keep in check and the infections that were becoming more frequent one could see that she was fading fast. It was really ironic that she had passed seven months from the time when she experienced her trauma. God had completed his work with her and her mission was complete. What a great mother and such a compassionate and caring individual that she was. We will all truly miss her.

May 13, 2007, the day before mother's day, our mother's funeral was today. I had the privilege of preaching her home going service in the church that our family had founded in our uncle's living room. She was one of the charter members and had sung in the choir, served on many boards and committees. She was a very faithful and hard-working member of our community also.

After the service I was sitting alone reviewing the last seven months and I thought about the last time I had spoken with mom. I was giving her some money and she was thanking me for it and was saying that I didn't have to do it. But for all the things that she had done for me it wasn't enough that I was giving her. I then asked her where my father was because you know if you give your mother some money you'd better have a little something for your dad. The next day she went into the coma that she never recovered from. The insulin that she used to control her diabetes had been increased to such a level that it caused her not to have enough glucose in her system and she went into the coma. The fact that she had to take the insulin to control her diabetes is what had caused the coma, but why did mother have diabetes?

Mother used to exercise a little bit but she had stopped. She didn't watch her diet and ate about whatever she wanted to. She was carrying more weight than she should have been. She was also on insulin for her diabetes & she had been a smoker, she had a heart condition and high blood pressure.

If mother were here right now she would ask me the question; why do you think I died, what happened to me? And I would tell her that there are four keys that will ensure that we will have a great chance of living a long life and have good health and physical fitness. After seeing your doctor and getting a physical before you began your program the keys are:

1. Get the right kind of rest, 6-8 hours of sleep per night.
2. Eat the right kinds of foods, fruits and vegetables and lean cuts of meat, chicken, fish, etc. limit your sweets and processed foods. Don't eat after 8:00 p.m.
3. Exercise 30 to 40 minutes per day, walking is great but whatever exercise you do make sure you use the big core muscles of your body.
4. Don't put substances in your body that are bad for you: cigarettes, drugs, the wrong kinds of foods, alcohol, etc.

Why are these steps so important? The reason why these steps are so important is as follows. If we don't get the right kind of rest we will feel tired and as if we need energy. We would need energy that we would normally get from resting, but because we did not get our proper rest we feel sluggish, tired and in need of energy. What do we do? We go to our next source of energy; we go get something to eat. But the problem is we're not tired from being hungry we are tired because of sleep deprivation or lack of rest.

So we eat the food in an attempt to supply the energy that we can only get from resting and not from eating. We end up eating more food than we want to because our energy demand, which is due to needing more rest, is not capable of being satisfied by eating more food. Because we have eaten more food than we should have, we are putting on extra calories that we do not need and we are still feeling listless and tired because we have not satisfied our need for rest or sleep. We cannot satisfy our need for sleep with our need for food energy.

So what do we do next? Because we are still tired and need to get some rest we end up going to sleep or what we commonly call going into a "food coma". Now this creates another problem because now we have all this extra food energy that we are laying down and going to sleep on that is being stored on our bodies. Instead of burning it off this extra food energy is being stored or is accumulating on our bodies as fat.

Often times we will eat the wrong kinds of food or too much of the right kinds of food in an attempt to satisfy an energy shortage that is due to sleep deprivation and not to being hungry. This is like trying to charge the battery of our cars by hooking them up to a banana or a watermelon and expecting it to get charged up and perform at optimum power. This cycle can be repeated over and over again until we have accumulated so much stored food energy or fat that we will begin to have the other related illnesses that come with obesity. Sugar diabetes, high blood pressure, arthritis, heart disease, cancer's and so many of the other diseases that we are susceptible to when we are obese.

Because of the diseases we may need to have the medications with their dangerous side effects that can cause us to have other physical problems. If we use other drugs, cigarettes, alcohol, cocaine, marijuana etc. we can cause ourselves many great physical problems and ailments that are inherent with the use of these drugs. When we take drugs we are basically committing slow motion suicide. If we continue in that lifestyle it is just like taking a bottle of rat poison and ingesting small amounts of it every day for years and years until it finally kills us. What a waste, what a waste, what a waste.

Studies have shown that exercise is so important because it allows us to make our bodies strong and healthy. It builds up our vital organs like our hearts and lungs; it burns up excess calories and reduces fat. In a new study in the Science News February 25 2006 edition, Dr. Mercola commented that recent research evidence suggests "exercise makes us smarter and can help us learn things easier." Exercise has also been shown to be beneficial in maintaining memory, easing pain, preventing strokes, controlling type 2 diabetes and treating depression. Exercise is just good for all of us mom.

And mother would say somebody needs to tell everybody about these four rules so they can live longer and healthier lives. Well mom I'm going to do what you asked me to do and tell everyone who will listen about these four rules, so that their families and their loved ones will not have to experience the pain and the heart ache that our family has experienced.

I want all the people with big butts and big guts to know that you can lose them by abiding by my four rules. You can do it because you are worth it. All of you that think you're too old, you're not too old "you're vintaged" and like a fine wine you're getting better with age. I want you to know that you can still do the best that you can. The devil is going to try to tell you that you can't do it but I know what's inside of you. The Bible says greater is he that is in me then he who is in the world. You have greatness inside of you and if you will abide by my four rules, have a little bit of dedication, commitment and discipline; you can do it! You can get it done and have some fun. Come Alive Now!!

If you don't have your health you don't have anything!! What price or amount of money would you pay to have good health? What would you do to have good health? Come on lets change our lives and come alive and make ourselves a promise that we will give our best to become the best that we can be. Why because we are worth it. We are worth it! We are worth it! Began to experience life on a more vibrant level! Come alive now, come alive now, come alive now! Don't waste another moment living beneath the level of excellance that you should be living at right now!! Come alive Now, Right Now Come Alive, Come Alive, Come Alive at 55!!!!!!

NOW! MAY THE VERY GOD OF PEACE HIMSELF SANCTIFY YOU WHOLLY; AND I PRAY GOD MAY YOUR WHOLE SPIRIT, SOUL AND BODY BE PRESERVED BLAMELESS UNTIL THE COMING OF OUR LORD JESUS CHRIST!!!

Your humble teacher in Christ,
Dr. M. D. Brown 1st.

After watching many of his friends, associates, loved ones and finally his mother pass away much too early from health related issues which could easily have been avoided. Dr. Brown has taken his 40 years of experience in the area of physical fitness, 24 years in full potential development and 18 years in ministry and has combined them in a book that will show you how to live on a new level of awareness, strength and power. This book will show you just how easy it is for us to address one of the most important areas of our existence and to take control of it with the discipline and will power necessary to function and achieve those goals and objectives that we thought were just so many past hopes and dreams. After reading this book you will truly know how to focus all of your energies and efforts in a way to maximize every opportunity and to achieve your full potential. Isn't it time that You Came "ALIVE" at 55? When we become more "Vintaged" or more "Seasoned" the tendency is to be told or to tell ourselves to slow down and to be placed on the shelf like an old relic or trophy. But I am here to tell you that even though you may be a little older, you are not "DEAD", you are not finished you are not through. As my grandpa used to say, I Ain't Done Yet" and neither are you. This book can be beneficial to anyone who would like to prepare themselves for a better spiritual, intellectual and physical life at any age. But it targets those of us known as the "baby boomers" and lets you know that the best is yet to come, especially physically. This book will inspire you to new heights and bigger and better accomplishments and will help you look the best you have in many, many, many years. This book will make you say,

"I am alive at 55"

If you live to be 110 years old, you are only half way there!!

WHAT ARE YOU GOING TO DO WITH THE NEXT 55 YEARS?

Email address: mbrown1@neo.rr.com
Webpage addresses: www.mdb1.com,
www.mdb1.org and myaimstore.com/drmdb1

Printed in the United States
201827BV00002B/184-1026/P